THE WOMEN'S
HEALTH PRODUCTS HANDBOOK

"An excellent guide to those drugstore items the friendly ads insist are 'Safe!' or 'New and Improved!' From diet pills, vitamins, contraceptives, douches and tampons, this well-written source offers documented analyses and a glossary on drugs, labels and herbal remedies. Everything you wanted to ask your pharmacist but were afraid to pronounce."

— *Los Angeles Times*

"Highly recommended. . . . A concise consumer guide filled with helpful, easy-to-use product charts, which list the products' active ingredients, possible side effects, and dosage forms."

— *Library Journal*

"A thoroughly documented guide to products relating to menstruation, birth control, weight control and vaginal health, including prescription and non-prescription products."

— *National Women's Health Network Newsletter*

"Sorting out myths from facts, the author surveys brand name products used in menstruation, contraception, nutrition, and dieting. She suggests some simple at-home tests to determine an item's suitability, and she identifies the benefits and risks (such as toxic shock syndrome) involved."

— *Booklist*

"Carol Ann Rinzler has written a good-sense health guide for women. . . . She explains which products can promote health, which are ineffective but harmless and which may cause more problems than they solve."

— *The Globe*

"Advertising for female hygiene and health-care products is a multi-million-dollar industry in the United States. But many of us don't know all the physical and psychological side effects of over-the-county devices and medications. Carol Ann Rinzler has solved this problem by compiling [this guide]. . . .

"Rinzler delivers it all with simple, easy-to-read explanations of female symptoms, plus charts describing the drugs and devices currently sold to relieve these problems.

"Travel and high-pressure executive jobs can lead to stress and strain. the pill-popping, alcoholic executive who works under pressure and suppresses rage gets little coverage. As women executives are emerging on the American business scene in significant numbers, they should welcome this handy health guide. . . .

"Women who work, as well as those who are full-time homemakers, will find [this guide] an excellent resource."

— *Working Woman*

"As Carol Ann Rinzler points out in this frank and charmingly informative book, most of us buy specific feminine products either because we like the packaging, have been impressed by the advertising, or have already used a product for years—without really knowing whether another product might work better. Rinzler's product guide is designed to answer questions women ask about the effectiveness, risks, and benefits, of health or hygiene products. . . .

"Drawing from sources like Consumer Reports, the Physicians' Desk Reference, the Merck Index, and industry and government reports, Rinzler pulls together a lot of information many women will be glad to find in one place. Her historical accounts of products such as menstrual pads are fascinating and her approach to each selection is sensible, amusing and woman-to-woman. . . .

"A specialized but useful book by a first-class writer on health care."

— *The Plain Dealer*

Praise for Carol Ann Rinzler's *Estrogen and Breast Cancer*

"Straight talk—informative and accessible—
about a health issue of concern to millions."

— *Kirkus*

"Rinzler assumes little and explains much. . . . Her balanced and
informative look at an ongoing problem may not solve it, but
Rinzler offers new thoughts and a comprehensive knowledge."

— *Publishers Weekly*

"Carol Rinzler has carefully documented the history of estrogen
and breast cancer. Every woman considering post-menopausal
hormonal therapy should read this book first and remember
that there is no free lunch."

— Susan M. Love, M.D., author of *Dr. Susan Love's Breast Book*

"A blistering indictment."

— *San Francisco Chronicle*

"*Estrogen and Breast Cancer* should be read by any woman
considering the birth control pill or hormone replacement therapy,
and by prescribing physicians."

— National Council on Women's Health

"If you are a woman who is using—or considering using—hormone
replacement therapy or oral contraceptives, or if you are someone
who is angry at officials for not committing the funds to finding a
'cure' for breast cancer, read this book."

— *Natural Health*

THE WOMEN'S HEALTH PRODUCTS HANDBOOK

Carol Ann Rinzler

Hunter House
PUBLISHERS

Library of Congress Cataloging-in-Publication Data
Rinzler, Carol Ann.
The Women's Health Products Handbook / Carol Ann Rinzler.
p. cm.
Includes bibliographical references and index.
ISBN 0-89703-210-2 (cloth). — ISBN 0-89793-209-9 (pbk.)
1. Women—Health and hygiene—Handbooks, manuals, etc.
2. Hygiene products—Handbooks, manuals, etc.
3. Health products—Handbooks, manuals, etc.   I. Title
RA778.R49   1996
613'.04244'0296—dc20   96-27095
CIP

Ordering
Hunter House books are available at bulk discounts for textbook/course adoptions; to qualifying community, healthcare, and government organizations; and for special promotions and fundraising. For details please contact:

Special Sales Department
Hunter House Inc., PO Box 2914, Alameda CA 94501-0914
Tel. (510) 865-5282 Fax (510) 865-4295
e-mail: marketing@hunterhouse.com

Individuals can order our books from most bookstores or by calling toll-free:
1-800-266-5592

Cover design: Jil Weil Designs, Oakland
Book design and production: Paul J Frindt
Project editor: Lisa E. Lee   Copy editor: Mali Apple
Editorial assistance: Kim A. Wallace, Jane E. Moore
Proofreader: Lee Rappold   Indexer: Kathy Talley-Jones
Marketing: Corrine M. Sahli   Promotion: Kim A. Wallace
Customer support: Sharon R. A. Olson, Edgar M. Estavilla, Jr.
Order fulfillment: A & A Quality Shipping Services
Publisher: Kiran S. Rana

Typeset in Arrus BT with tiles in Lithograph by Hunter House Inc.
Printed and bound by Publishers Press, Salt Lake City, UT
Manufactured in the United States of America

9 8 7 6 5 4 3 2 1   Second revised edition

LIST OF CONTENTS

LIST OF CONTENTS (CONT'D)

LIST OF TABLES

LIST OF TABLES (CONT'D)

IMPORTANT NOTE

The ideas, procedures, and suggestions in this book are not intended to be a substitute for consulting with your physician. All matters regarding your health require medical supervision. In addition, the fact that some ingredients or products are described as causing allergic reactions, irritation, or other side effects does not mean that these side effects will occur in every person who uses these products or every time these products are used.

This book contains a number of charts comparing products. While every effort has been made to obtain a representative sampling of products, these charts may not include every product in a given category. Inclusion of a product in a chart does not imply an endorsement; omission does not imply a criticism.

Most of the ingredients and label claims noted in the charts are from product packages or inserts that were available in New York City in the summer of 1995 or from interviews with manufacturers in the spring of 1995. A few of the products mentioned were introduced since 1995. Always check the label: while every effort has been made to verify ingredients, some may have been added or omitted since this book was written. All prices shown were obtained in one discount drugstore in New York City; they are for comparison purposes only and may be higher or lower than prices for the same product in other stores or other parts of the United States. Please note that many of the product names listed in this book are trademarked.

COMMON ABBREVIATIONS

FDA	=	Food and Drug Administration; the federal agency charged with monitoring the safety and effectiveness of foods, drugs, and cosmetics
OTC	=	over-the-counter; a term used to describe drugs available without a prescription
g	=	gram; a unit of mass equal to 1,000 milligrams or 1,000,000 micrograms. 28 grams = 1 ounce.
mg	=	milligram; 1/1,000th of a gram; 1,000 micrograms
mcg	=	microgram; 1/1,000,000th of a gram; 1/1,000 of a milligram
l or L	=	liter; a unit of volume equal to 10 deciliters or 1,000 milliliters. 1 liter = 1.056688 quarts = 33.8 ounces.
dL	=	deciliter; 1/10th of a liter
ml	=	milliliter; 1/1,000th of a liter

FOREWORD

These days, almost everyone buys drugs in large discount stores or supermarkets. The number of choices—once you find the right aisle—is astonishing. But increasing media coverage of the side effects of drugs and other health products has made people more skeptical of advertising claims. Many physicians are overwhelmed by requests for information concerning the safety, usefulness, and cost effectiveness of various women's health products. The questions are varied: do I need vitamin supplementation; how safe are liquid dieting agents; is douching helpful or harmful; is it safe to use tampons?

With so many products to choose from and with such high-powered marketing and advertising skills being used to sell them, we're more inclined to ask which products are most necessary and effective. Given our increasing understanding of the complex nature of drugs, it is not surprising that consumers have questions about how to use them safely.

How adequate are the responses of doctors, nurse practitioners, physician assistants, and health educators in both conventional settings and the newer HMOs, PPOs, Ambulatory Care Clinics, and so on? Although many of the "report cards" of managed care facilities show that most patients are satisfied with their treatments, what about the information they receive? Are patients aware of things like the effects of over-the-counter medications?

There is no answer yet. What we do know is that over 50 percent of patients take *prescription* medications incorrectly. This has resulted in the FDA requiring pharmacists to give verbal and written information to their customers when then they fill prescriptions. It also confirms the need for a consumers' guide to products that are not regulated.

Now it is no longer uncommon for the consumer to want to be able to evaluate a prescription or "over-the-counter" product. And today she can easily do so—provided she has an understanding of the major evaluation criteria and the necessary product information. This book provides both and brings to the subject a degree of clarity and rationality rarely seen elsewhere.

Carol Ann Rinzler is very direct in her explanations of unexpected responses, interactions with other drugs, and the side effects of over-the-counter products. Effects of megadoses, common misusages, and most important of all, warnings of toxicities, are stressed in each section. She points out things that ought to be but are not common knowledge, such as the effectiveness of the morning-after pill in preventing pregnancy, and other forms of emergency contraception that are currently available.

I think copies of this book should be in the waiting rooms of all medical clinics and physicians' offices, as well as in the lounges and libraries of every high school and college in the nation. The information in *The Women's Health Products Handbook* is vital for consumers. This clear and concise resource will help you stay in good health.

Marcia L. Storch, M.D.
Scientific and Medical Director of the American
Menopause Foundation and Obstetrician/Gynecologist
practicing at Women to Women in Yarmouth, ME.

CHAPTER 1

VAGINAL HEALTH AND HYGIENE

Is there any one of us who has not experienced a sudden, paralyzing fear that a lover will find our genitals unattractive or even downright offensive?

Probably not. The suggestion that the vagina is ugly or smelly seems to be something all women run into at some time in their lives. Perhaps it surfaces when we first begin to menstruate and learn about the need for hygiene during our periods. Maybe we get the idea from our friends or from a boyfriend who tries to prove his sophistication with an offhand remark about our sexuality or our bodies.

Either way, the result is that many of us occasionally yearn for a deodorized, sanitized, desexualized vagina. Of course, we are nudged along in this by advertising for douches and sprays and powders and cleansers that claim to cure a problem that, it turns out, isn't really a problem at all.

DOUCHES

In normal circumstances, the healthy vagina is never "dirty." Like your eyes, nose, mouth, and throat, your vagina is lined with tissues called *mucous membranes* that produce sticky secretions (mucus). These secretions are natural cleansers that wash away internal surface debris such as dead cells.

Obviously, you need to maintain a daily relationship with soap and water to wash the external surfaces of the vaginal folds where secretions and perspiration collect and are digested by bacteria that excrete odorous compounds. If you do not bathe or shower every day, the discharge may accumulate on the external surface of the vaginal folds and produce an odor.

Other causes of vaginal odor include semen, blood from menstruation, infections, and foreign objects such as tampons that have been left in the vagina. In addition, colonies of resident "friendly" bacteria—a mixture of bacteria that maintain the normal acid pH of the vagina and that fight off hostile invading pathogens—may cause the vagina to give off an odor.

The normal scent of the healthy vagina is neither unpleasant nor unclean. In fact, like the natural scent of male sweat, the scent of the vagina is an erotic attractant. Most over-the-counter (OTC) douches, therefore, are simple cosmetics whose main purpose is to flush out the vagina.

WHAT'S IN AN OTC DOUCHE

OTC douches come in two varieties, medicated and nonmedicated. The medicated products, to be used only at a doctor's direction, are designed to relieve itching and irritation due to a minor vaginal infection. A nonmedicated douche's only raison d'être is to flush out the vagina and make it feel or smell "nicer" and, presumably, more attractive to a sexual partner.

A commercial douche may contain as many as 10 or 11 ingredients. While that may seem high to anyone used to douching with a simple homemade solution of vinegar and water, the list of chemicals permitted in OTC douches has actually shrunk considerably over the past 20 years following a continuing series of reports from Food and Drug Administration panels created specifically to rate the safety and effectiveness of ingredients in OTC products. For example, 15 years ago, OTC douches might contain the antimicrobials hexachlorophene and a variety of phenol compounds, which could be absorbed into the body through the vaginal walls. Today, these substances have been banned from douches and many other OTC products.

ANTIMICROBIALS   are supposed to eliminate organisms that cause odors and itching. Medicated douches, such as BETADINE M.D., BIDETTE, MASSENGILL, SUMMER'S EVE, or YEAST GARD (medicated), contain povidone-iodine in a concentration sufficiently strong to relieve minor vaginal irritations. But the concentrations of other potential antimicrobials in nonmedicated OTC douches, such as cetylpyridinium chloride or boric acid, are so weak that these ingredients function not as antiseptics but as surfactants or preservatives (see below).

SURFACTANTS OR DETERGENTS   such as octoxynol-9 or sodium lauryl sulfate reduce surface tension, the tendency for molecules in a liquid to cling to each other. Surfactants (short for *surface active agents*) are chemicals that reduce the electrical charges that hold molecules together so that a liquid can spread out more quickly to coat a surface. Surfactants are also *mucolytic,* meaning that they break up mucus. These two properties—the ability to keep molecules from clinging together and the ability to break up mucus—make surfactants efficient detergents (cleansers). Adding a surfactant to a douche makes the douche solution more effective at washing secretions out of the vagina. The downside is that all surfactants can be drying if used too often.

ACIDIFIERS AND ALKALIZERS   promise to alter the pH (acid/base balance) of the vagina so as to encourage the growth of protective bacteria normally living there or to increase the cleansing power of the douche. "Friendly" microbes flourish in an acid environment, so a basic (alkaline) solution cleans better. Acetic acid (the active ingredient in vinegar), citric acid, lactic acid, and monobasic sodium phosphate are used to acidify vaginal douches. Baking soda (sodium bicarbonate), a natural detergent, makes douches more alkaline.

The decision whether or not to use an acid or basic douche can be a delicate one. First, there is no evidence to show that swishing either an acid or a basic solution in and out of the vagina has any lasting effect on the internal pH. Second, the acids and bases in premixed OTC douches are in dilute concentrations so that they are unlikely to cause irritation. Thus, they are also unlikely to have any real effect and are generally considered harmless.

As a general rule, if you are using a douche in the absence of disease simply to feel "fresh," an acidic douche, which reinforces the natural acidity of the vagina, is the better choice. If you are douching to eliminate secretions, an alkaline douche is a more effective detergent.

PERFUMES   (read "fragrance" on the label) can mask odors for a short time but are potential irritants, allergens, and allergic sensitizers (substances that make you sensitive to other chemicals). As a general rule, washing daily with soap and water is a more effective way to clean the external vaginal area, removing secretions and sweat that resident microbes can convert to odoriferous compounds.

COLORING AGENTS   such as D&C Red #28 or FD&C Blue #1*

---

* D = drugs, C = cosmetics, F = food. A coloring agent labeled D&C may be used only in products to be used externally; a coloring agent labeled FD&C may be used in foods as well as in drugs and cosmetics that may be swallowed (for example, mouthwash).

make a douche look appealing (translation: "fresh" or "cool"), but that's about all. Colors serve no useful function, and they are potential allergens.

PRESERVATIVES   inhibit the growth of molds and bacteria, keeping products from deteriorating on the drugstore shelf or in your medicine cabinet. Benzoic acid, methylparaben, and propylparaben are used as preservatives in douches. Low concentrations of potential antimicrobials such as cetylpyridinium chloride and boric acid also serve as preservatives. *Sequestrants* such as disodium EDTA protect the freshness and safety of a douche solution because they attract and inactivate metal ions that bacteria and other microbes need to live.

Douches also contain *thickeners* such as SD alcohol 40 to make the product feel smoother and *emulsifiers* such as dibasic sodium phosphate to prevent mixtures of oils and water from separating.

THE RISKS AND BENEFITS OF DOUCHING

As cosmetics, OTC douches are a wash-out and an expensive one at that. If you do not have a vaginal infection or a sexually transmitted disease or an allergic reaction and if you are not taking birth control pills (which sometimes trigger a copious flow of vaginal secretions), your vagina is perfectly capable of cleaning itself.

The ingredients in OTC douches are so dilute that the solutions are neither harmful nor particularly helpful. As one physician on the Food and Drug Administration advisory panel (originally convened in the 1970s to reevaluate vaginal drug products) put it, the concentrations of ingredients in the products are so weak and are in the vagina for such a short time that they cannot be either very effective or very harmful unless they are used more often than the manufacturers' directions suggest or are used in a homemade solution mixed too strong. According to the American Pharmaceutical Association, homemade vinegar-and-water douches should not be stronger than 2 tablespoons vinegar to 1 quart water.

Bathing daily will remove secretions and perspiration from the outer vaginal area, preventing the bacteria that live there from turning them into odorous compounds. As you might expect, there is a study to back this up. In 1965, researchers asked a group of women with vaginitis to gently wash their vaginal and anal areas each day with warm water and mild soap. The result? About 94 percent of the women who followed the regimen effectively relieved the symptoms of vaginitis; only 5 percent had recurrent symptoms.

DOUCHING SAFELY

What, you may logically ask, can possibly go wrong when I use a product whose ingredients are pleasing but so weak that practically everyone agrees they are innocuous?

That's a reasonable question. Here's a reasonable answer: What's wrong with douching may not be the ingredients in the product but the act of douching itself.

DOUCHING INSTEAD OF VISITING THE DOCTOR   Many of us douche to get rid of an annoying discharge. Some discharges, such as the slippery mucus that accompanies ovulation, are completely natural; they do not indicate disease. Others, such as the increase in secretion that may come with using birth control pills, are annoying but harmless. But infections also cause discharges. It can be difficult to identify infections from a discharge, as some are accompanied by itching and burning sensations, and others are not. Diagnosing the causes of these symptoms can require expert advice, maybe even a laboratory test. In any event, self-medication with a douche is risky. It may spread the infection so that by the time you are miserable enough to schedule an appointment, you are facing a raging case of heaven-knows-what that would have been easier to treat at the start. Finally, never douche before a doctor's appointment. You don't have anything she hasn't seen before, and seeing what you do have is an important part of the examination.

DOUCHING TOO OFTEN   Before we can say what may happen if you douche too often, we have to define what "too often" means. It's not easy. Some gynecologists say that if you have no medical problems requiring a douche, any douching is too much and too often. Others say that if the douche solution is not medicated, and properly diluted, neither too acid nor too alkaline, it does not matter how often we douche. Others opt for a modified middle: once a week.

Douching too frequently increases the risk of allergic reactions. It may also be irritating to the vaginal tissues, flushing out natural lubricating secretions so effectively that you end up with the internal equivalent of dishpan hands. In addition, excessive washing of the vagina may alter the pH so that the friendly bacteria cannot thrive. Their absence clears the way for pathogens to multiply unchecked, a reaction similar to what can follow long-term use of antibiotics.

There's more. It is possible that frequent douching may spread vaginal infections past the cervix into the uterus. Some studies have shown a link between frequent douching and a higher risk of pelvic inflammatory disease (PID) and salpingitis (an inflammation of the fallopian tubes), perhaps because the constant internal bathing dissolves the protective mucus plug generally found at the opening of the cervix. In one study of women admitted to Yale–New Haven Hospital clinics, nearly two-thirds of the women with PID or salpingitis were in the habit of douching once a week or more compared with less than 20 percent of the control group.

DOUCHING TOO ROUGHLY   No matter how often reproductive and urinary organs are referred to as "plumbing," what is down there is living tissue, not copper or plastic drainpipe. To protect the tissue, experts (including the Food and Drug Administration advisory panel on contraceptives and other vaginal drug products) recommend a number of simple, commonsense rules.

First, insert the douche nozzle very gently to avoid bruising the walls of the vagina or bladder, the latter a particular danger if you are sitting upright on the toilet while you douche. This is a convenient position for douching, but it shortens the vagina and moves the bladder forward—a position more likely to be hit by the nozzle. Do not exert force to insert the nozzle. A tightening of the muscles around the entrance to the vagina is the usual reason women have difficulty using a douche. This reaction, usually a result of simple tension, may happen at any time, to anyone, even women who have been using a douche successfully for years. The muscles may relax if you just sit quietly for a few minutes. If there is no change, do not force the nozzle into the vagina. Simply forget about douching, at least for the moment. If the same reaction occurs repeatedly, you may want to check with your doctor the next time you go for a pelvic examination to be certain there is no organic problem.

If you use a homemade douche solution, be sure that it is sufficiently diluted so as not to be irritating to the vaginal tissues. If you use a commercial product, follow the directions to the letter. Premixed solutions are already the right concentration; medicated solutions have precise measured amounts to be mixed. Do not vary this formula. If you use your own solution or are required to add water to prepare a commercial product, use warm (not hot) water.

Be careful not to send the liquid into the vagina under pressure. It is not necessary to whoosh the liquid in and out to get the best results. In fact, if the solution flows in under pressure, it may be forced up past the cervix, increasing the risk of PID or salpingitis. It is easier to control the flow from a fountain syringe (a douche bag plus plastic tubing and a nozzle) than from a bulb syringe (a squeezable plastic container attached directly to a nozzle). With a bulb syringe, you must squeeze the bulb to get the solution up and out, so it is already being forced out of the container under pressure. With a fountain syringe, however, it is possible to vary the pressure by raising or lowering the bag slightly. The most effective position seems to be sitting on the toilet, facing the back, with the nozzle inserted into the vagina and the bag held just above your waist, so that gravity pulls the liquid down into the vagina and right out again. Never hold the lips of the vagina closed while you are douching, as this may force liquid up past the cervix.

When you finish douching, throw out a disposable douche package; wash and dry reusable equipment. The American Pharmaceutical Association recommends boiling douche equipment to sterilize it; check the package or with the manufacturer to be certain your douche bag, tubing, and nozzle can be boiled safely.

Never use your douche equipment as an enema bag; that can spread organisms from anus to vagina. And never use an enema nozzle for douching. The single opening at the tip of the enema nozzle delivers too forceful a stream of liquid; you need the gentle spray you get from the multi-opening douche nozzle.

DOUCHING FOR CONTRACEPTION   A douche is not a contraceptive. Even if you were to break all speed records for human runners, by the time you insert the douche solution into the vagina, sperm are already on their way to the cervix and some may already be into the uterus. In addition, if you use a spermicide or a diaphragm and spermicide, using a douche soon after intercourse will wash the jelly, cream, foam, or dissolved tablet or suppository right out of your vagina, seriously compromising their ability to protect you against pregnancy. As for that archetypal homemade supposed-contraceptive douche, a bottle of carbonated soda, it's worthless—and downright dangerous. Soda is carbonated, containing oxygen and carbon dioxide gases. When it enters the vagina under pressure, the liquid is forced through the cervix into the uterus which, unlike the stomach, is lined with tiny, open blood vessels. Theoretically, the gases in the soda will enter the blood vessels, perhaps even sending a fatal oxygen bubble (an embolism) into the bloodstream.

DOUCHING WHILE PREGNANT   You can sum up all the rules about douching while pregnant in two words: better not. While a woman is pregnant, the number of blood vessels in the lining of the uterus increases, as does the risk of forcing air past the cervix while douching. (See the soda warning above.) In addition, douching during pregnancy may spread a vaginal infection from mother to fetus, expose the fetus to a whole shelf full of chemicals, and increase the risk of rupturing the membrane surrounding the fetus.

VAGINAL INSERTS

NORFORMS are small, waxy suppositories designed to "deodorize" the vagina. The ingredients are similar to what is found in a douche: an acidifier, antiseptic, surfactants, emulsifiers, and a preservative to protect the mixture from microbial contamination. BETADINE medicated suppositories also promise to deodorize vaginal tissues, but they are "medicated" with povidone-iodine, an antiseptic for minor itch or irritation. There is no evidence that either of these products is more cleansing or deodorizing than daily bathing.

VAGINAL SPRAYS

There is nothing so simple and useless that someone with a little imagination cannot complicate and make profitable. Douches at least have a function to justify their existence: they do flush out the vagina. But what can we say about the vaginal spray except that it exists solely to spritz a layer of perfume or fragrant powder on top of any vaginal secretions or perspiration lying around on the outer vaginal surface?

First introduced in 1966, vaginal deodorant sprays (a.k.a. feminine hygiene sprays) were an overnight sensation. Within five years, there were more than 30 brands on the market, and enough aerosols were being aimed at American vaginas to account for sales totaling more than $67 million.

But then, you might say, the spray hit the fan. In 1972, when the Food and Drug Administration banned hexachlorophene from use in any OTC product, the sprays lost their only active ingredient, an antiseptic supposed to eliminate odor-causing bacteria. The FDA struck again in 1975, prohibiting manufacturers from using the word "hygiene" in brand names, packaging, or advertising for vaginal sprays because, they said, the product had absolutely no medical or hygienic activity, not even the ability to get rid of odors. About all they could do, critics said, was produce side effects.

In the early 1970s, reactions to vaginal sprays were practically a medical growth industry. Women turned up regularly at their gynecologists' offices with itchy, reddened skin, infections, or swollen labia (the external folds of the vagina). If they used the sprays right before intercourse (which probably seemed like a good thing to do with a product that promised to make your private parts smell good) or used them to create homemade deodorant tampons, also a hot new item in the early 1970s, the ingredients—perfumes, antiseptics, propellants— were pushed inside the vagina. When that happened, women were not alone in their misery. Male partners of women who had spritzed before sex were likely to wake up the next morning complaining of itchy, reddened skin on the penis.

WHAT'S IN A VAGINAL SPRAY?

Many of the symptoms associated with the early sprays were caused by antiseptics. When the antiseptics were eliminated, reports of reactions decreased. But what's left may also be irritating or allergenic. In addition to fragrance, vaginal sprays usually contain a propellant, one or more emollients, a solvent, and perhaps a powder as a thickener.

PROPELLANTS   are the most prominent ingredient in any aerosol spray, including those meant for the vaginal area. Propellants such as isobutane are not allergenic but can be intensely irritating. If you hold the spray too close to the vagina, the propellants may chill or freeze the moist membranes, or cause swelling and inflammation.

EMOLLIENTS   such as isopropyl myristate, lanolin, and mineral oil are oily substances that make a liquid spray feel rich, even soothing, to the skin. Lanolin is the only allergen in the group, but all three are easily digested by bacteria. Paradoxically, these anti-odor sprays may actually increase bacterial conversion of sweat and secretions into odorous compounds.

SOLVENTS   such as SD alcohol 40 dissolve the solid ingredients in the product to make a solution that can be sprayed on the skin.

USING SPRAYS SAFELY

To avoid injury while using a vaginal spray, hold the spray at least 8 inches from your body. Never aim it directly at the vaginal opening. Never spray a tampon and then insert it. The ingredients are meant for external use; they will irritate vaginal mucous membranes.

If you experience any reaction to the spray, stop using it immediately and check with your doctor.

FEMININE WASHES

Feminine washes are liquid detergents similar to other liquid skin soaps. This means that while they will certainly perform as promised, they are no more (or less) effective than bathing with your usual soap and water or with a liquid soap such as IVORY SKIN CLEANSING LIQUI-GEL.

As long as you are not sensitive to an ingredient in the soap, both feminine washes and liquid soaps are considered safe. But there are two simple cautions. First, never use a feminine wash or liquid soap as a douche or to make a bubble bath. Neither type of cleanser has been tested or approved for use on internal tissues. Second, never substitute a shampoo or dishwashing liquid for a liquid skin cleanser. Dishwashing products contain bleaches and brighteners, and their detergents are more concentrated. Shampoos, too, have more concentrated cleaning ingredients and may contain ingredients such as colors and antidandruff agents that are safe to use on small areas but not over the entire body.

PREMOISTENED TOWELETTES

One reason vaginal infections are so common is that bacteria and yeast love the moist, warm environment of the vagina. Anything that increases the natural warm moistness—for example, pantyhose, nylon underpants, or tight-fitting jeans—also increases the risk of playing host to these microbes.

One objection to premoistened "feminine towelettes" is that if we use them too often, the skin stays damp and vulnerable. However, if we use these individually wrapped wipes only once in while, they

FEMININE WASH VERSUS LIQUID SOAP: CAN YOU TELL THEM APART?	
Product 1	*Product 2*
Water, sodium laureth sulfate, sodium lauryl sulfate, lauramide DEA, sodium sulfate, cocomidopropyl betaine, sodium chloride, fragrance, tetrasodium EDTA, citric acid	Water, sodium laureth sulfate, magnesium laureth sulfate, sodium laureth-8 sulfate, sodium oleth sulfate, magnesium oleth sulfate, fragrance, DMDM, hydantoin, laurimidopropyl betaine, myristamine oxide, lactic acid, PEG 120, methyl glucose dioleate, fragrance, sodium methylparaben, sodium ethylparaben, sodium propylparaben, methylchoroiso-thiazolinone, methyliso-thiazonolone, D&C Red #33
Product 1 is IVORY LIQUI-GEL.	Product 2 is MASSENGILL FEMININE WASH.
Source: Products on sale in New York City, summer 1995.	

are handy for sponging off vaginal secretions or menstrual fluid that has spilled off a pad or past a tampon when we are away from home and cannot bathe immediately.

The ingredients in the liquid on the towelettes are similar to those in douches and vaginal sprays. If you are sensitive to one product, you may be sensitive to another.

FEMININE POWDERS

Body powders are used to soothe, or to dry an area by soaking up moisture. Talc, once used as a base in virtually all dusting powders, has been eliminated from vaginal products because its use around the vaginal area may be linked to ovarian cancer.

In place of talc, feminine powders use cornstarch. They may also contain anticaking agents (tricalcium phosphate) or antistatic agents (benzethonium chloride) to keep the powder from clumping, coloring

COMPARING TALC-FREE CORNSTARCH POWDERS
IS THE SPECIAL PRODUCT WORTH THE PRICE?

Product (Supplier)	Price & Size	Price per oz.
SUMMER'S EVE feminine powder (Personal Laboratories/C.B. Fleet)	$2.99 7 oz.	43¢
VAGISIL feminine powder (Combe)	$2.59 7 oz.	37¢
JOHNSON'S pure cornstarch baby powder (Johnson & Johnson)	$3.69 22 oz.	17¢
MEXANA medicated (Schering Plough)	$3.79 11 oz.	34¢
ARGO CORNSTARCH	$1.26 16 oz.	8¢

Source: Products on sale in New York City, summer 1995.

agents (magnesium stearate/white), emollients or skin soothers (aloe, mineral oil), an adsorbent to keep the powder on the skin (silica), and fragrance.

In the late 1980s, a number of researchers suggested that using talc powders in the genital area might increase the risk of ovarian cancer. While this remains to be proven, feminine powders now use cornstarch rather than talc, as do several brands of bath powder such as JOHNSON'S BABY POWDER (PURE CORNSTARCH),* which contains cornstarch plus fragrance and an anticaking agent (tricalcium phosphate), or the somewhat more complex MEXANA MEDICATED, which contains cornstarch plus fragrance, whiteners (zinc oxide, kaolin), an antistatic agent (benzethonium chloride) to keep the powder from clumping, a preservative (camphor), and an antiseptic (eucalyptus oil).

See pages 13–16 for a comparison of OTC cleansing products.

---

* Do not confuse this product with the original formula JOHNSON'S BABY POWDER, which contains talc.

COMPARING OTC CLEANSING PRODUCTS

Product (Supplier)	Ingredients—Features
DOUCHES	
BETADINE M.D. (Purdue Frederick)	povidone-iodine, fragrance; to be mixed with water in douche bag — concentrate
BIDETTE BAKING SODA (Clinipad)	sanitized water, sodium bicarbonate (baking soda), diazolidinyl urea, disodium EDTA — disposable, pre-mixed
BIDETTE MEDICATED (Clinipad)	povidone-iodine, sanitized water — disposable; concentrate
BIDETTE VINEGAR AND WATER (Clinipad)	vinegar, water, sorbic acid — disposable, pre-mixed
MASSENGILL DOUCHE POWDER (SmithKline Beecham)	sodium chloride, ammonium alum, PEG 8, phenol, methyl salicylate, eucalyptus oil, menthol, thymol, D&C Yellow #10, FD&C Yellow #6 — concentrate, to be mixed in douche bag
MASSENGILL BABY POWDER (SmithKline Beecham)	water, SD alcohol 40, lactic acid, sodium lactate, octoxynol-9, cetyl pyridinium chloride, propylene glycol, diazolidinyl urea, methylparaben, propylparaben, disodium EDTA, fragrance, FD&C Blue #1 — disposable, pre-mixed
MASSENGILL BAKING SODA (SmithKline Beecham)	sanitized water, sodium bicarbonate (baking soda) — disposable, pre-mixed
MASSENGILL COUNTRY FLOWERS (SmithKline Beecham)	water, SD alcohol 40, lactic acid, octoxynol-9, cetyl pyridinium chloride, propylene glycol, diazolidinyl urea, methylparaben, propylparaben, disodium EDTA, fragrance, D&C Red #28, D&C Blue #1 — disposable, pre-mixed
MASSENGILL MEDICATED (SmithKline Beecham)	povidone-iodine, sanitized water — disposable, concentrate

Product (Supplier)	Ingredients—Features
MASSENGILL VINEGAR AND WATER (SmithKline Beecham)	*"extra mild"*: water, vinegar *"extra cleansing"*: water, vinegar, cetyl pyridinium chloride, diazolidinyl urea, disodium EDTA — disposable, pre-mixed
SPECIFICS ALOE VERA (Lake Pharmaceuticals)	aloe vera, water, lactic acid, sodium benzoate, docusate sodium — disposable, pre-mixed
SPECIFICS HERBAL VINEGAR & WATER (Lake Pharmaceuticals)	purified water, white vinegar, octoxynol-9, sorbic acid, fragrance — disposable, pre-mixed
SUMMER'S EVE POSTMENSTRUAL (Personal Laboratories/C.B.Fleet)	purified water, sodium chloride, dibasic sodium phosphate, methylparaben, disodium EDTA, monobasic sodium phosphate, sodium lauryl sulfate, propyl paraben — disposable, pre-mixed
SUMMER'S EVE MEDICATED (Personal Laboratories/C.B.Fleet)	povidone-iodine — concentrate
SUMMER'S EVE VINEGAR AND WATER (Personal Laboratories/C.B. Fleet)	purified water, vinegar, benzoic acid — disposable, pre-mixed
YEAST GARD MEDICATED (Women's Health Institute/Lake Pharmaceuticals)	octoxynol-9, purified water, lactic acid, sodium lactate, sodium benzoate, aloe vera — disposable, pre-mixed
VAGINAL INSERTS	
BETADINE MEDICATED SUPPOSITORIES (Purdue Frederick)	povidone-iodine in propylene glycol base
NORFORMS (C.B. Fleet)	PEG-18, PEG-32, PEG-20 stearate, benzethonium chloride, methylparaben, lactic acid
VAGINAL SPRAYS	
BIDETTE MIST (Clinipad)	isobutane, SD alcohol 40, isopropyl myristate, fragrance

Product (Supplier)	Ingredients—Features
FDS/with powder FEMININE DEODORANT SPRAY (Alberto Culver)	"baby powder" and "extra strength": Isobutane, isopropyl myristate, cornstarch, mineral oil, fragrance, lanolin alcohol, hydrolyzed silica, magnesium stearate, benzyl alcohol
FEMININE WASHES	
MASSENGILL (SmithKline Beecham)	water, sodium laureth sulfate, magnesium laureth sulfate, sodium laureth-8 sulfate, sodium oleth sulfate, magnesium oleth sulfate, laurimidopropyl betaine, myristamine oxide, lactic acid, PEG 120, methyl glucose dioleate, fragrance, sodium methylparaben, sodium ethylparaben, sodium propylparaben, methyl-choroisothiazolinone, methyl-isothiazolinone, D&C Red #33
SUMMER'S EVE (Personal Laboratories/C.B. Fleet)	purified water, ammonium laureth sulfate, cocoamidopropylamine oxide, PEG-75 lanolin, phosphoric acid, PEG 120, methyl glucose dioleate, disodium EDTA, fragrance, methylchoroisothiazolinone, FD&C Blue #1, methylisothiazolinone
PREMOISTENED TOWELETTES	
BIDETTE FEMININE CLOTH TOWELETTES (Clinipad)	water, SD alcohol 40-B, polysorbate 20, benzthonium chloride, propylparaben, menthol, sodium bicarbonate, fragrance — individually wrapped
MASSENGILL soft cloth towelette (SmithKline Beecham)	*Unscented:* water, octoxynol-9, lactic acid, sodium lactate, potassium sorbate, disodium EDTA, cetylpyri-chloride *Baby powder scent:* water, lactic acid, potassium sorbate, octoxynol-9, disodium EDTA, cetylpyridinium chloride, fragrance — individually wrapped

Product (Supplier)	Ingredients—Features
PREPARATION H CLEANSING TISSUES (Whitehall)	purified water, propylene glycol, phenoxyethanol, methylparaben, propylparaben, butylparaben, citric acid
SUMMER'S EVE INTIMATE CLEANSING CLOTHS (Personal Laboratories/C.B. Fleet)	purified water, octoxynol-9, sodium benzoate, fragrance, citric acid, disodium EDTA — individually wrapped
TUCKS TAKE ALONG premoistened hemorrhoidal/vaginal pads (Warner Welcome)	witch hazel, water, glycerin, alcohol, propylene glycol, water, sodium citrate, diazolidinyl urea, citric acid, methylparaben, aloe vera gel, propylparaben — individually wrapped
FEMININE POWDERS	
SUMMER'S EVE (Personal Laboratories/C.B. Fleet)	cornstarch, tricalcium phosphate, octoxynol-9, fragrance
VAGISIL (Combe)	cornstarch, aloe, magnesium stearate, silica, benzethonium chloride

Sources: Products on sale in New York City, summer 1995. Donald R. Miller and Mary Kuzel, "Personal care products," *Handbook of Nonprescription Drugs,* 9th ed. (Washington, DC: American Pharmaceutical Association, 1990). Colgate-Palmolive consumer information, 1-800-255-7552. Proctor & Gamble consumer information, 1-800-633-9758.

VAGINAL ITCH

If there is anything more common than the common cold, it is the common itch.

Skin is composed of three layers of cells: the epidermis (the top, outer layer of dead cells), the dermis, and the deep dermis. When the deep dermis is pierced, we feel a solid, aching pain. When the dermis is hit, the pain is sharper, like a pinprick. But when the sensation reaches only the epidermis—as when the skin is very dry—we feel something annoying but too mild to be called pain. That's an itch.

All itches are annoying. Some may be maddening. But for sheer emotional impact, so long as they do not signal serious disease, none quite measures up to an itch in the crotch.

It's not just that polite society tends to frown on our scratching away at our privates in public (thus denying us a handy remedy for a sudden, fleeting itch). It's also the suspicion that whatever is making us itch is not, well, *nice*. No matter how removed we may be from our grandmothers' white gloves and lace, the fact is that none of us faces a vaginal itch with aplomb.

PHYSIOLOGY OF AN ITCH

We itch when we're bitten by an insect, such as a mosquito, that injects a protein under the skin, triggering a histamine reaction. We itch when we are exposed to allergens such as poison ivy or poison oak; these are also histamine reactions. Eating a food to which we are allergic can set off an itchy rash, or hives. So can emotional stress, which also causes itching without a rash. Anemia, diabetes, and dry skin can make you itch. Nonstop itching all over the body may be an early warning sign of leukemia, Hodgkin's disease, cancer of the liver, or pancreatic cancer. Sometimes, simply thinking about itching is enough to make us scratch.

We instinctively try to relieve an itch by substituting pain. We scratch. We call up time-tested home remedies such as ice cubes on mosquito bites or hot compresses on hives. By applying heat or cold to the skin, we may overload the nerve endings so that they blank out for a while and "forget" to tell us we're itching.

PRODUCTS FOR VAGINAL ITCHING

An itch is a symptom, not a disease. To eliminate it, we need to get rid of whatever is causing it. The most common causes of itches in the vaginal area are irritations (your pants are too tight and they rub) and allergic reactions to a cosmetic drug, fungus, or bugs. You may also itch from a discharge caused by a vaginal infection (see page 30) or very dry vaginal tissues (see page 24).

Because there are many reasons why you may develop an itch in the genital area, it is imperative to know why you're itching before you medicate. This is particularly true now that drugs formerly sold only by prescription are available over-the-counter.

Caution: Read all labels carefully. If the label does not say that the product can be used in the external vaginal/anal area, do not use it to relieve a vaginal itch.

ANESTHETIC ANTI-ITCH CREAMS   VAGISIL and YEAST GARD are water-based creams that wash off easily and will not stain clothes. They each contain a topical anesthetic (benzocaine) as well as a mild antibacterial (resorcinol). They also work in the anal area, male or female, to relieve mild itching from hemorrhoids. Benzocaine, a popular ingredient in OTC products such as sunburn creams and sprays, sore-throat lozenges, and hemorrhoid products, works by numbing surfaces to which it is applied. Resorcinol is mildly effective against some organisms that cause vaginitis (see table, pages 21–22).

These products are safe as long as you follow the directions on the package, applying them only to external surfaces. Both benzocaine and resorcinol can trigger allergic reactions—some itchy. Using benzocaine may sensitize you to sulfa drugs; resorcinol can dry and irritate your skin.

But the principal risk of vaginal anti-itch products is that they may mask symptoms requiring medical treatment. All packages carry warnings to stop using the product if an itch worsens or lasts longer than a few days, but it is always safer to assume that any itch lasting long enough to send you to the drugstore in search of relief has already gone on too long. No benzocaine or resorcinol product will cure a bacterial or fungal infection, and it may complicate or worsen an allergic reaction.

ANTI-INFLAMMATORY CREAMS AND OINTMENTS   The active ingredient in CALDECORT, CORTAID, CORTIZONE, LANACORT-10, and

other anti-inflammatory products is hydrocortisone, a steroid that reduces swelling and alleviates the itching of allergic reactions. Once
sold only by prescription, hydrocortisone was approved for sale as an
OTC drug in 1980 when manufacturers were able to show that it was
safe even when applied to the skin in strong concentrations.

Nonetheless, it still pays to use hydrocortisone products cau-
tiously. What makes them so effective against allergic reactions is their
ability to suppress the natural defensive reactions of the immune system. Therefore, if you apply a hydrocortisone product to a bacterial,
viral, or fungus infection, the infection may quickly spread.

Read all labels carefully to be certain that the products are meant
to be used in the genital area. For example, SOLARCAINE and LANA-
CAINE, which effectively relieve the pain and discomfort of minor
burns or sunburn, and BENADRYL, which relieves minor itch, are not
formulated for use in the vaginal area.

ANTIFUNGAL DRUGS   The fungus most commonly found in the
genital area is *Tinea cruris*, better known as "jock itch." A rashy misery
that in a truly egalitarian world might also be known as the pantyhose
plague, *Tinea* does not play favorites, gender-wise. It thrives in any
warm, damp, airless groin, so drying thoroughly after bathing and
wearing cotton panties or pantyhose with a cotton crotch or loose
jeans or slacks often prevents Tinea from taking hold.

The most effective nonprescription antifungal drug is tolnaftate,
the active ingredient in AFTATE, TINACTIN, and TING. Undecylenic
acid, calcium undecylenate, and zinc undecylenate, the active ingredi-
ent(s) in CALDESENE, CRUEX, and DESENEX, and hydroxyquinoline
(AMMENS MEDICATED) also prevent fungi from reproducing and thus
will eventually cure an itch. Tolnaftate, the undecylenates, and hydroxyquinoline are non-irritating and rarely cause an allergic reaction.
Hydroxyquinoline has a characteristic mild saffron-like odor; the undecylenates, some say, smell like urine or sweat, an odor masked by
fragrance in the product. Clotrimazole and miconazole, two highly effective drugs found in OTC products for yeast infections (see tables,
pages 32–34), are also useful against fungi.

When a *Tinea* infection persists or worsens, doctors may order
the prescription drug griseofulvin (FULVICIN, GRIFULVIN V, GRISACTIN,
GRIS-PEG). Taken orally, griseofulvin is deposited primarily in skin,
hair, and nails, where it interrupts fungal reproduction, preventing
fungi from multiplying. Griseofulvin makes estrogen less effective; if
you are taking birth control pills, you must switch to another form of

contraception. If you are pregnant or suspect you may be, tell your doctor. Although human studies are not available, griseofulvin is known to cause birth defects in the offspring of laboratory animals given the drug while pregnant.

INSECTICIDES   Bugs? Us? Could be. We may like to think that *Phthirus pubis* (the crab louse, commonly known as "crabs") and the "itch mite" (*Sarcoptes scabies*) only happen to other people, but nobody told the bugs. As they have since the beginning of time, they continue to hop from one warm body to another without checking pedigrees.

Crab lice are parasites that look like teensy crabs. They do not survive on smooth skin, preferring to run around in hairy places such as the head and groin. In fact, if you look closely, you can actually see them tracking along through the underbrush as it were, their eggs just tiny bumps on the base of each hair. They are acquired through intimate contact with infested furniture, bedclothes, and people. Itch mites burrow into the skin around hair follicles. They are acquired by skin-to-skin contact with an infected person. If you are the infested party, common courtesy dictates that you inform your intimate partners. If anyone in your house has either bug, *everyone* should be treated.

The best-known OTC drug for crabs is RID, a shampoo containing pyrethrins, natural insecticides from plants. RID also comes in a spray to be used on furniture and bedding. The drawback: If you have hay fever, you may be allergic to RID. Scabies is treated with the prescription drug cromiton (EURAX), which is available as a cream.

The charts on pages 21–23 compare a selection of anti-itch products on the market.

COMPARING THE PRODUCTS: OTC ANTI-ITCH PREPARATIONS

Product	Form	Active Ingredients	Features
CREAMS/OINTMENTS			
CALDECORT, CALDECORT LIGHT (Ciba)	cream	hydrocortisone (anti-itch, anti-inflammatory)	fragrance-free
CALDESENE (Ciba)	ointment	calcium undecylenate (antibacterial, antifungal)	may have unpleasant odor, like sweat; fragrance
CRUEX (Ciba)	cream	undecylenic acid, zinc undecylenate (antibacterial, antifungal)	may have unpleasant odor, like sweat; fragrance
CORTAID (Upjohn)	cream, ointment	hydrocortisone (anti-itch, anti-inflammatory)	fragrance-free
CORTIZONE-5, CORTIZONE-10 (Thompson Medical)	cream, ointment	hydrocortisone (anti-itch, anti-inflammatory)	fragrance-free
DESENEX AF Prescription strength (CIBA)	cream	clotrimazole	fragrance-free
LANACORT 10 (Combe)	cream	hydrocortisone acetate (anti-itch, anti-inflammatory)	fragrance
TINACTIN JOCK ITCH (Schering Plough)	cream	tolnaftate (antifungal)	fragrance-free
TING (Ciba)	cream	tolnaftate (antifungal)	fragrance-free
VAGISIL (Combe)	cream	benzocaine (topical anesthetic), resorcinol	

Product	Form	Active Ingredients	Features
VAGISIL MAXIMUM STRENGTH (Combe)	cream	benzocaine (topical anesthetic), resorcinol	
YEAST GARD (Lake Pharmaceuticals)	cream	benzocaine (topical anesthetic), resorcinol	
POWDERS			
AFTATE (Schering Plough)	aerosol powder	tolnaftate (antifungal)	contains talc
AMMENS (Bristol Myers)	powder	hydroxyquinoline (antifungal, antiperspirant)	contains fragrance; talc-free
CALDECORT (Ciba)	spray powder	hydrocortisone (anti-itch, anti-inflammatory)	fragrance-free
CALDESENE (Ciba)	shaker	calcium undecylenate (antibacterial, antifungal)	may have unpleasant odor, like sweat; fragrance; talc
CRUEX (Ciba)	shaker	calcium undecylenate (antibacterial, antifungal)	may have unpleasant odor, like sweat; fragrance; talc
CRUEX (Ciba)	spray powder	undecylenic acid, zinc undecylenate (antibacterial, antifungal)	may have unpleasant odor, like sweat; fragrance; talc
DESENEX AF Prescription strength (Ciba)	spray powder	miconazole	fragrance-free, talc-free

Product	Form	Active Ingredients	Features
GOLD BOND (Martin Himmel)	powder	menthol (local anesthetic), zinc oxide (antiseptic), boric acid* (antifungal) * Not listed as an active ingredient	contains talc; and eucalyptol, thymol, and methyl salicylate, potentially irritating aromatic oils that serve as perfumes, antiseptics, and counter-irritants
TINACTIN JOCK ITCH (Schering Plough)	spray powder	tolnaftate (antifungal)	fragrance-free, contains talc
TING (Ciba)	shaker, spray powder	tolnaftate (antifungal)	powder contains talc
SPRAY LIQUIDS			
AFTATE (Schering Plough)	aerosol liquid	tolnaftate (antifungal)	
DESENEX AF Prescription strength (Ciba)	spray liquid	miconazole	fragrance-free
TING (Ciba)	spray liquid	tolnaftate (antifungal)	

Sources: Products on sale in New York City, summer 1995. *Physicians' Desk Reference for Nonprescription Drugs,* 16th ed. (Montvale, NJ: Medical Economics Data, 1995).

VAGINAL LUBRICANTS AND MOISTURIZERS

Like the lining of the mouth, eyes, nose, and throat, the lining of the vagina is normally moist with mucous secretions that protect and cleanse the tissues. A sudden increase in vaginal secretions is an important characteristic of sexual arousal, designed to make intercourse easy and comfortable.

Vaginal dryness, a lack of sufficient secretions, affects about 40 million American women, either temporarily or permanently. The most common cause of vaginal dryness is the natural decline in estrogen secretion at menopause. Before menopause, women may experience estrogen-related vaginal dryness after delivery when estrogen levels recede from a pregnancy high; while breastfeeding when prolactin, the hormone that triggers milk production, suppresses estrogen secretion; or after surgical removal of the ovaries. Danazol (DANOCRINE), a synthetic hormone used to treat endometriosis, and tamoxifen (NOLVADEX), an anti-estrogen used in the treatment of breast cancer, also suppress estrogen and may dry the vaginal lining. Antihistamines and tricyclic antidepressants such as amitriptyline (ELAVIL) reduce the secretions from all mucous membranes, including the vagina. Finally, tension or stress may short-circuit sexual response, including natural lubrication of the vagina.

Vaginal dryness is uncomfortable and sometimes itchy, and increases the risk of infection, irritation, and injury during sex. For women whose dryness is temporary, lubricated condoms provide relief. Others may find that applying spermicidal jelly in the vagina, or smoothing it onto a condom or the penis, does the trick. The heavier, slicker *vaginal lubricants* such as K-Y JELLY, LUBRIN, MAXILUBE, and TOUCH provide more effective relief. These lubricants are designed to make the walls of the vagina slippery for short periods of time. They may be used with condoms, but they do not protect against sexually transmitted disease and they are not contraceptives. They should never be used in place of a spermicidal gel, jelly, or cream.

A second type of product, *vaginal moisturizers* such as GYNE-MOSTRIN, MOIST AGAIN, and REPLENS, employ more advanced technology, using chemicals whose molecules attract and hold water against the vaginal surface, sometimes for 24 hours or longer. Vaginal lubricants are meant for women of any age; vaginal moisturizers were created primarily for postmenopausal women who need long-term moisturizing but do not wish to use estrogen replacement therapy.

COMPARING THE PRODUCTS:
VAGINAL LUBRICANTS & MOISTURIZERS

Product	Category	Ingredients	Features
GYNE-MOISTRIN (Schering Plough)	moisturizer (gel)	polyglyceryl-methacrylate, water, propylene glycol, methylparaben, propylparaben	forms lattice on vaginal walls that holds moisture and releases it over time; apply before intercourse; may be used with a condom
K-Y JELLY (Johnson & Johnson)	lubricant (jelly)	chlorhexidine gluconate, glucano delta lactone, glycerin, hydroxyethyl-cellulose, methylparaben, purified water, sodium hydroxide	apply before intercourse; may be used with a condom
LUBRIN (Upsher-Smith)	lubricant (suppository)	capyrlic/capric triglyceride, laureth 23	apply before intercourse; may be used with a condom
MAXILUBE (Mission)	lubricant (jelly)	silicon oil, glycerin, carbomer 934, triethanolamine, sodium lauryl sulfate, parabens	apply before intercourse; presumed not to harm condoms

Product	Category	Ingredients	Features
MOIST AGAIN (Lake Consumer Products)	moisturizer (gel)	water, carbomer, glycerin, triethanolamine, aloe vera, citric acid, chlorhexidine glutamate, sodium benzoate, potassium sorbate, diazolidinyl urea, sorbic acid	
REALITY (Wisconsin Pharmacal)	lubricant	water, glycerin, sodium carboxy-methyl-cellulose, EDTA, methylparaben, polysorbate 80, propyl paraben	sold in packet with REALITY female condom
REPLENS (Warner Lambert)	moisturizer (gel)	purified water, mineral oil, glycerin, polycarbophil, carbomer 934P, hydrogenated palm oil, glyceride, sorbic acid	molecules hold 60 times their weight in water; attach by binding to cells in vaginal wall; hold moisture in place for 24 hours or more; packed in individual applicators; apply 2–3 times a week
TOUCH Personal lubricant (London International/ Schmid)	lubricant	water, propylene glycol, hydroxy-ethyl-cellulose, benzoic acid, sodium hydroxide	

Sources: Products on sale in New York City, summer 1995. *Physicans' Desk Reference for Nonprescription Drugs,* 16th ed. (Montvale, NJ: Medical Economics Data, 1995).

ESTROGEN

The most effective vaginal lubricant for postmenopausal women is estrogen, given as a pill, via a transdermal patch on the skin (trans = across, dermal = skin), or applied as a cream. However, the hormone's benefits are shadowed by its risks.

RISKS AND BENEFITS   Estrogen supporters contend that it reduces the risk of heart disease and osteoporosis, but many researchers question whether the protection estrogen affords is truly significant.

Contrary to popular belief, not every older woman is at risk of osteoporosis. Furthermore, a 1995 analysis by the American College of Physicians, reported in the *Harvard Women's Health Watch,* showed that taking hormone replacement therapy reduces a 50-year-old woman's risk of hip fracture by only 2 to 3 percent, from slightly more than 15 percent to a bit less than 13 percent. Among black women in this country, osteoporosis is so rare that, the newsletter said, the "preventive effects of HRT* are insignificant."

As for heart disease, no randomly selected study has ever conclusively proven estrogen's benefits for large groups of women. As the Harvard letter notes, only 12 percent of all postmenopausal women may avoid heart attack by taking estrogen alone; if they are taking estrogen plus progestins, the rate drops between 7 and 12 percent.

On the other hand, taking estrogen raises a woman's risk of blood clots. If taken during pregnancy, it can harm a developing fetus, and it is a reproductive carcinogen.

Using estrogen at menopause increases a woman's lifetime risk of endometrial cancer by more than 800 percent. Unlike ordinary endometrial cancers, the ones linked to estrogen therapy are aggressive and often fatal. Adding progestin to the estrogen reduces the risk of endometrial cancer. In 1995, following a number of deaths among volunteers in the hormone replacement trials at the National Institutes of Health's program called Women's Health Initiative, NIH ruled that no woman with an intact uterus who enters the study would receive estrogen alone.

Estrogen raises a woman's risk of fatal ovarian cancer. On May 1, 1995, the American Cancer Society released new data from its Cancer Prevention Study II, a prospective mortality survey of more than 240,000 women, showing that women who take estrogen for at least

---

* hormone replacement therapy = estrogen plus progestin

six years at menopause have a risk of fatal ovarian cancer 40 percent higher than women who have never taken hormones. At 11 years' use, the risk is 70 percent higher for women taking estrogen. There is no information on whether adding a progestin to the estrogen reduces this risk.

Estrogen puts a woman at risk of breast cancer. Between August 1976 and June 1995, more than 26 studies here and abroad have demonstrated a consistent statistical link between hormone replacement therapy and increased risk of breast cancer. Reducing the dose makes no difference; neither does adding progestins. Women who take hormones at menopause increase their risk of breast cancer from 30 to 700 percent, depending on how long they use hormones and their own personal risk factors.

There are two kinds of estrogen used in therapy for human beings: natural estrogens and synthetic estrogens. *Conjugated estrogens* are a mixture of estrogens obtained from the urine of pregnant mares including estradiol, estrone, and equilin. *Esterified estrogens* are a mixture of estrogenic substances, principally estrone, which is excreted by pregnant mares. *Estradiol* is the primary estrogen secreted by the human ovary. *Estrone* is a less-active metabolite of estradiol, found in the urine of pregnant women and mares. *Estropipate* is a form of estrone. *Quinestrol* is a synthetic estrogen similar to ethynyl estradiol, used in birth control pills. There is no proof that synthetic estrogens are more or less hazardous than natural estrogens.

The chart on the following page describes a selection of ERT products on the market.

COMPARING THE PRODUCTS:
ESTROGEN REPLACEMENT THERAPY (ERT)*

Product (Supplier)	Active Ingredient	Form
ESTRACE (Mead Johnson)	estradiol	tablets
ESTRADERM (Ciba)	estradiol	transdermal patch
ESTRATAB (Solvay)	esterfied estrogens	tablets
ESTRATEST (Solvay)	esterfied estrogens	tablets
ESTROVIS (Parke-Davis)	quinestrol	tablets
MENEST (SmithKline Beecham)	esterfied estrogens	tablets
OGEN (Abbott)	estrone	tablets, cream
OGEN (Abbott)	estropipate	tablets, cream
ORTH-EST (Ortho)	estropipate	tablets
PREMARIN (Wyeth-Ayerst)	conjugated estrogens	tablets, cream

* Hormone replacement therapy (HRT) is estrogen plus a progestin. PREMPRO, introduced by Wyeth-Ayerst in 1995, provides 2 tablets a day, a PREMARIN tablet and a tablet containing the progestin medroxyprogesterone acetate (MPA). PREMPHASE, also introduced by Wyeth Ayerst in 1995, provides 28 PREMARIN tablets, with 14 progestin tablets to be taken during the second half of the cycle, days 14 to 28.

Sources: Physicians' Desk Reference, 48th ed. (Montvale, NJ: Medical Economics Data, 1994). PREMPRO/PREMPHASE introductory advertising, Wyeth-Ayerst, 1995.

PRODUCTS FOR VAGINAL INFECTIONS

Vaginitis isn't one disease. It is a catchall term for a collection of infections caused by various organisms, many of which cause itchy, smelly, or irritating discharges. Some can be transmitted during sex. Some infections can be prevented by simple hygiene, such as washing before intercourse. Most require a laboratory test to determine exactly which organism is to blame, and most should be treated with prescription drugs. And, if one partner is treated, the other should at least be seen by a doctor, and probably treated to avoid passing the infection back and forth or to another sexual partner.

The most common vaginal infection is caused by a yeast organism, *Candida albicans* (monilia), that normally lives in the vagina in perfect balance with other microbes. However, when something happens to weaken the bacteria population and upset the balance, *Candida* begins to multiply out of control, producing a white, lumpy discharge sometimes described as resembling cottage cheese. Yeast infections are common among women taking antibiotics. Using birth control pills also increases the risk of yeast infection because they make the vaginal environment less acidic and therefore less hospitable for resident bacteria.

PRESCRIPTION DRUGS FOR YEAST INFECTIONS

Nystatin is the grand old lady of drugs for *Candida* infections. It was discovered in 1950 by two biochemists, Rachel Brown and Elizabeth L. Hazen, who named it in honor of New York State (they were both working in the New York State Department of Health at the time). Nystatin—available alone (MYCOSTATIN) or in a combination product (MYTREX) containing the anti-inflammatory steroid triamcinolone acetonide—is the kind of drug doctors, researchers, and patients dream about. It works. It has been around for some time, which means we have the best possible evidence—patient use—to prove that it is safe and effective. It usually relieves the symptoms of *Candida* within three days; applications continue until the infection is cured.

Butaconazole (FEMSTAT), ketoconazole (NIZORAL), terconazole (TERAZOL), and ketoconazole (NIZORAL) are related to clotrimazole and miconazole. All are as effective as vaginal creams against *Candida*; ketoconazole and terconazole may also be useful against other fungi. All may cause local itching and allergic reactions.

The newest and most powerful drug against vaginal yeast infections is fluconazole (DIFLUCAN), the first of a new class of broad-spectrum antifungal drugs. Fluconazole, which damages yeast and fungal cell walls and inhibits the cells' ability to process steroid chemicals such as cholesterol and estrogen, cures yeast infections by preventing the cells from growing and replicating themselves.

Fluconazole was introduced as a treatment for *Candida* infections of the mouth, throat and esophagus, and urinary tract, as well as bacterial meningitis. It also seems to cure vaginal yeast infections with one 150-mg tablet in one day. This regimen, approved by the FDA in 1994, is relatively inexpensive (about $10). The most common side effects—nausea, cramping, and diarrhea—appear to be mild and short-lived, although they do occur more frequently with fluconazole than with the OTC drugs clotrimazole and miconazole.

But this is not the whole picture. If you are sensitive to the antifungal, antiyeast drugs clotrimazole and miconazole, you may also be sensitive to fluconazole. If you use fluconazole for recurrent yeast infections, you may become resistant to the drug. Taking fluconazole increases the effects of anti-asthma drugs, anticoagulants, diabetes medication, and drugs used to suppress rejection in transplant patients. It alters the body's metabolism of the hormones in birth control pills. Taking the tuberculosis drug rifampin along with fluconazole makes the latter less effective. Like ketoconazole, fluconazole has been associated, although rarely, with three serious adverse reactions: liver poisoning, anaphylactic shock, and exfoliative dermatitis, a potentially fatal condition in which the skin literally peels off. Finally, although there are no adequate controlled studies for human beings, fluconazole is known to cause spontaneous abortion in pregnant rabbits and severe fetal bone defects in rats, reactions also observed with terconazole.

For a comparison of antiyeast products see the chart on pages 32–34.

COMPARING THE PRODUCTS: ANTIYEAST PREPARATIONS

Product	Form	Ingredients	Features
OTC VAGINAL CREAMS			
FEMSTAT 3 (Proctor & Gamble)	cream	butoconazole	3 applications; requires only 3 days' use
GYNE-LOTRIMIN (Schering Plough)	cream	clotrimazole	packed with tube of cream and reusable applicator *or* cream plus 7 disposable applicators *or* 7 prefilled disposable applicators; fragrance-free
MONISTAT-7 (Ortho)	cream	miconazole	greaseless; does not stain clothes; sold in package with 7 prefilled, disposable applicators
MYCELEX-7 (Miles)	cream	clotrimazole	greaseless; does not stain clothes; sold in tube with reusable applicator *or* in package with 7 disposable applicators; fragrance-free

Product	Form	Ingredients	Features
OTC VAGINAL INSERTS			
GYNE-LOTRIMIN (Schering Plough)	inserts	clotrimazole	sold in package with 7 inserts plus applicator *or* 7 inserts, applicator, and GYNE-LOTRIMIN cream; fragrance-free
MONISTAT-3 (Ortho)	inserts	clotrimazole	3 inserts plus applicaor and cream; oil in inserts may weaken condoms
MONISTAT-7	inserts	miconazole	7 inserts
MYCELEX-7 (Miles)	inserts	clotrimazole	sold in package with 7 inserts and an applicator *or* with 7 inserts, an applicator, and a tube of MYCELEX-7 cream; greaseless and nonstaining; fragrance-free
VAGISIL YEAST CONTROL, homeopathic (Combe)	suppositories	pulsitilla, Candida, parapsilosis, Candida albicans	homeopathically prepared to 28X; fragrance-free
PRESCRIPTION PRODUCTS			
FEMSTAT (Syntex)	cream	butaconazole	cream for 3 days available in prefilled applicators
DIFLUCAN (Pfizer)	oral tablet	fluconazole	one dose (150 mg)

Product	Form	Ingredients	Features
NIZORAL (Janssen)	cream	ketoconazole	once a day for 2 weeks
TERAZOL 3 (Ortho)	vaginal suppository, cream	terconazole	1 suppository a day for 3 days *or* cream once a day for 3 days
TERAZOL 7 (Ortho)	cream	terconazole	once a day for 7 days
MYCOSTATIN (Bristol Myers)	vaginal tablets, cream, ointment	nystatin*	once a day for 3 days to relieve symptoms, 14 days for cure
MYTREX (Savage)	cream, ointment	nystatin, triamcinolone acetonide	once a day for 3 days to relieve symptoms, 14 days for cure

* Nystatin is also available as a generic drug.

Sources: Products on sale in New York City, summer 1995. DIFLUCAN advertisement/package insert, July 1994. Donald R. Miller and Mary Kuzel, "Personal care products," *Handbook of Nonprescription Drugs,* 9th ed. (Washington, DC: American Pharmaceutical Association, 1990). *The Merck Manual,* 16th ed. (Rahway, NJ: Merck Research Laboratories, 1992). *Physicians' Desk Reference for Nonprescription Drugs,* 16th ed. (Montvale, NJ: Medical Economics Data, 1995). Ruth Winter, *A Consumer's Dictionary of Cosmetic Ingredients* (New York: Crown Publishers, 1994).

OTC ANTIYEAST PRODUCTS

Recently, the FDA reclassified the prescription drugs clotrimazole and miconazole as OTC products. The first is available in a variety of greaseless, nonstaining creams and vaginal inserts (GYNE-LOTRIMIN, MYCELEX 7); the second, as a cream (MONISTAT 7).

Both clotrimazole and miconazole are effective against *Tinea cruris* (jock itch) as well as yeast infections; both are likely to work within a week; both may cause skin reactions (blistering, peeling, itching, burning, or reddening); both may be absorbed through the vagina; neither has been proven safe during the first trimester of pregnancy.

While switching these drugs from prescription to OTC made it more convenient to treat yeast infections, it also places a serious responsibility on the consumer to be cautious when using OTC antiyeast products. In particular:

1. *Don't self-diagnose.* If this is the first time you have had a vaginal discharge, itch, or irritation, see your doctor before starting treatment. You want to be certain your problem is really a yeast infection.

2. *Never use an OTC product for a foul-smelling vaginal discharge.* A smelly, colored discharge may indicate a more serious infection.

3. *If you don't get better quick, see your doctor.* A yeast infection should respond within a week. If yours doesn't, you may have a medical condition such as pregnancy or diabetes that increases your susceptibility to yeast infections. Ditto for an infection that recurs within 2 or 3 weeks.

4. *Exposed to HIV? See your doctor.* If you have been exposed to HIV, the virus associated with AIDS, and are having recurrent vaginal infections, your immune system may have been compromised. Curing the yeast infection may require a different treatment plan.

5. *Pregnant? Check with your doctor.* Never use an OTC antiyeast product when you are pregnant except with your doctor's advice.

FOLK MEDICINE FOR YEAST INFECTIONS

The healthy vagina is home to many friendly bacteria including some remarkably similar to the *Lactobacilli,* bacteria that turn milk into yogurt. When we take antibiotics, these bacteria are destroyed, and yeast organisms flourish. It seems logical to think that if we can get more "good" bacteria into the vaginal area or nourish the ones still alive there, they will once again come into their own, establish a healthy balance, and decimate the unfriendly yeasts.

One way to enrich the vaginal environment is to add *acidophilus* bacteria, the bacteria in yogurt. Many women who are taking antibiotics add yogurt to their diet or—going a more direct route—smear yogurt on the vaginal area or douche with yogurt or a yogurt culture, available from health food stores. Waste of time, said much of the medical establishment. Messy, said many of the rest of us.

Then in 1992, a small study at the Long Island Jewish Medical Center in New Hyde Park, New York, followed 13 women as they first regularly consumed yogurt containing *Lactobacillus acidophilus* and then when they did not. The results, published in *The Annals of Internal Medicine,* showed that the acidophilus yogurt was so effective at preventing yeast infections that the women refused to give it up for the second part of the study.

DRUGS USED TO TREAT NON-YEAST VAGINAL INFECTIONS

Trichomonas vaginalis (sometimes called *Trich,* pronounced *trick*) is a protozoan, a one-celled parasite that lives in the vagina and male urethra. Sexual partners may pass it back and forth during intercourse, or it may be picked up from a contaminated toilet or towel. Regardless of how we acquire it, *Trich* can remain in the vagina for long periods of time without causing any problems. Approximately one in five women will develop a *Trich* infection at some point during her reproductive years. The infection produces a smelly, frothy, dark discharge, variously described as green, gray, or brown. The vagina is itchy and irritated, sometimes so sensitive that intercourse is painful. A pain higher up in the pelvis suggests that the infection has moved into the uterus.

The treatment of choice for *Trich* and another organism, *gardnerella* is metronidazole (FLAGYL) injection, gel, or vaginal inserts, prescribed either as one relatively large single dose or in smaller doses for 7 days. Though laboratory studies show metronidazole to cause cancer in mice and possibly rats, there is no evidence that it is a human carcinogen. There is some evidence that *Trich* may respond to clotrimazole, the active ingredient in several OTC medications and anti-yeast products.

Bacterial infections such as *chlamydia, mycoplasma,* and *E. coli* produce a grayish smelly discharge, which is itchy and irritating. These infections are treated with doxycycline (DORYX, VIBRAMYCIN, VIBRA-TABS), an antibiotic related to tetracycline. The most common viral infection, genital herpes, is treated with acyclovir (ZOVIRAX). As of this writing, acyclovir is available only by prescription, but the FDA is reviewing the possibility of making it a nonprescription product. Acyclovir's adverse effects may include a change in menstrual cycle and flow, skin rash, acne, hair loss, an upset stomach, and joint and muscle pain.

SOURCES

Boston Women's Health Book Collective, *The New Our Bodies, Ourselves* (New York: Simon and Schuster, Touchstone, 1992).

Colgate-Palmolive consumer information, 1-800-255-7552.

Current Medical Diagnosis and Treatment 1993, Lawrence M. Tierney Jr., et al., eds. (Norwalk, CT: Appleton and Lange, 1993).

"Folk remedy seems to help fight vaginal yeast infections," *New York Times,* March 10, 1992.

Harrison's Principles of Internal Medicine, 12th ed., Jean D. Wilson, et al., eds. (New York: McGraw-Hill, 1991).

Harvard Women's Health Letter, May 1995.

Jacobs, Michael R., and Paul Zanowiak, "Topical anti-infective products," *Handbook of Nonprescription Drugs,* 9th ed. (Washington, DC: American Pharmaceutical Association, 1990).

Long, James W., and James J. Rybacki, *The Essential Guide to Prescription Drugs* (New York: Harper Collins, 1995).

The Merck Index, 11th ed., Susan Budavari, ed. (Rahway, NJ: Merck & Co., 1989).

The Merck Manual, 16th ed., Robert Berkow, ed. (Rahway, NJ: Merck Research Laboratories, 1992).

Miller, Donald R., and Mary Kuzel, "Personal care products," *Hand-*

book of Nonprescription Drugs, 9th ed. (Washington, DC: American Pharmaceutical Association, 1990).

O'Connell, Mary Beth, "Vaginal dryness," *U.S. Pharmacist,* September 1994.

Physician's Desk Reference for Nonprescription Drugs, 16th ed. (Montvale, NJ: Medical Economics Data, 1995).

Physician's Desk Reference, 48th ed. (Montvale, NJ: Medical Economics Data, 1994).

Proctor & Gamble consumer information, 1-800-633-9758.

Smith, Anthony, *The Body* (New York: Viking Penguin, 1986).

Winter, Ruth, *A Consumer's Dictionary of Cosmetic Ingredients,* 4th ed. (New York: Crown Publishers, 1994).

CHAPTER 2

MENSTRUATION

MENSTRUAL PADS

From the beginning of time, or at least since women first began to use material to absorb menstrual fluid, women have been using one kind of pad or another—leaves, grass, or natural woven fibers such as washable cotton rags (the source of the slang expression "on the rag").

This kind of menstrual protection was so simple and effective that nobody thought to improve it until late in the nineteenth century when an American company, Johnson & Johnson, introduced LISTER'S TOWELS, disposable gauze-covered cotton pads. The towels were a genuine breakthrough and way ahead of their time. With public modesty in full Victorian flower, there was no way to advertise the new product, and after a while they simply disappeared.

World War I changed all that. In combat, battlefield medics used bandages made of cellulose rather than the customary cotton fabric. A natural fiber derived from wood pulp, cellulose is extraordinarily absorbent and, the nurses soon discovered, the perfect material for menstrual pads. In 1920, two years after the war ended, Kimberly-Clark, the paper company, introduced the first pad. KOTEX was a gauze-covered cellulose pad with long tabs to pin or hook it onto an elastic "sanitary belt."*

Unfortunately, magazines still refused to carry ads for such an intimate product, and many stores refused to display them. Nonetheless, the pads began to gain popularity and soon Johnson & Johnson introduced a second brand, MODESS. Although some women here and

---

* Menstrual pads are commonly described as "sanitary napkins," a somewhat offensive term that seems to imply that the women who use them (or the purpose for which they use them) are unsanitary. "Feminine napkins," a later euphemism, is confusing and essentially meaningless. The term "menstrual pad" is precise, descriptive, and nonjudgmental.

in Europe continued to use the old-fashioned washable cotton cloths, the new pads eventually became the predominant form of menstrual protection.*

THE MODERN MENSTRUAL PAD

Modern technology has improved the original product. The end tabs have been superseded by adhesive strips on the underside of the pad. Rayon fibers, also derived from wood, add absorbency to the core, protecting without adding bulk. A plastic shield on the bottom stops leaks; it works best when it continues up over the sides of the pad. To reduce spillage caused by the pad's shifting inside the panties, some pads are anchored with "wings" or "tabs" that fold under the sides of the pants. Additionally, some pantyliners and larger pads have "channels," shallow grooves in the pad's surface, to stop any overflow.

CHAFING   Women who dislike menstrual pads because they chafe the sensitive skin on the inside of the upper thighs may be more comfortable with a *slender* (narrower) pad or with a *shaped* or *contoured* pad that is wider at the ends and narrower through the middle.

DRYNESS   Next to chafing, a feeling of constant dampness next to your skin may be the most annoying aspect of using a menstrual pad. The modern menstrual pad is a sandwich, with a plastic shield on the bottom, a middle layer of absorbent material (usually cellulose), and a top wrap of synthetic material designed to draw liquid in toward the center of the pad so that the surface next to your body stays as dry as possible. The wrapper may feel like plastic (sometimes described as *dry weave*) or cloth (sometimes described as *cottony soft*). They work equally well, but some independent tests suggest that the ALWAYS pads may stay drier than most others. Try a few brands to see which works best for you. You probably need different sizes for different days. Of course, regardless of which pads you choose, it is important to change them as often as needed. This not only keeps you dry; it also prevents odors that develop when menstrual fluid is exposed to air. Some pads contain baking soda to neutralize these odors, but changing pads frequently is safer and more effective.

---

*   Washable, reusable cloth pads are still available from a number of companies in this country including Glad Rags, P.O. Box 12751, Portland, OR 97208, and New Cycle Products, P.O. Box 1775, Sebastopol, CA 95473.

POTENTIAL SIDE EFFECTS   While easy to use, menstrual pads are not free of side effects. The pad itself provides a pathway along which bacteria can move between the vaginal and anal areas. If you have a vaginal discharge, a pad rubbing against the external vaginal tissues may worsen the irritation and discomfort. In addition, the perfume in scented pads can be irritating and allergenic.

CHEMICAL HAZARDS   The cellulose in menstrual pads is made from wood pulp commonly bleached with chlorine. In the bleaching process, dioxins are created. Some studies show that exposure to dioxins increases the risk of cancer. Although there is no evidence linking the dioxins in menstrual pads to an increased risk of any type of cancer, some women prefer pads made without chlorine-bleached fibers. The alternative is a pad made from cellulose that comes from wood pulp bleached with hydrogen peroxide. Two such brands, NATRACARE and SEVENTH GENERATION, are both available in health food stores.*

CHOOSING A MENSTRUAL PAD

The perfect menstrual pad is best defined by what it does not do. It doesn't chafe, it doesn't rub, it doesn't leak, and it doesn't shift inside your underpants.

Modern pads come in a variety of sizes to match the menstrual flow, which starts light, is usually heaviest on the second or third day, and then tapers off. There are currently no FDA standards for menstrual pads, but for convenience, it is logical to divide them into six basic categories: panty-liners, ultra-thin maxipads, thin maxipads, regular maxipads, extra-protection pads, and maximum-protection pads.

PANTYLINERS   First introduced by Kimberly Clark (LIGHTDAYS) in 1975, these are very flat pads designed for use on days when the menstrual flow is very light. They can also be used to protect against vaginal discharge.

Basic, straight-sided pantyliners such as ALWAYS and CAREFREE come in regular length (about 6 1/2") and "long" (about 7 1/2"), plain

---

* If your store does not stock these brands, you may contact the companies: Natracare, 191 University Boulevard, Denver, CO 80206 (800-796-2872); and Seventh Generation, 49 Hercules Drive, Colchester, VT 05446 (802-655-6777).

or "deodorant" (with baking powder or a dusting powder scent). AL-
WAYS CONTOURS and LIGHT DAYS COMFORT DESIGN are wide at the
ends and narrow in the middle; LIGHT DAYS OVALS are, well, oval.

The surface of the pad may be flat or quilted; some (ALWAYS
SHEER CONFIDENCE, ESSENTIALS ULTRA DRY) are slightly more puffy,
and thus more absorbent, than others. The grooves along the sides of
ESSENTIALS WITH CHANNELS may offer extra protection against spills.
LIGHT DAYS WRAPAROUNDS (regular and long) have wings. Most pan-
tyliners (including the chlorine-free SEVENTH GENERATION) except NA-
TRACARE have a plastic shield on the bottom.

ULTRA-THIN MAXIPADS   These are full-size pads, approximately
8 1/2" by 2 1/2" overall (the absorbent pad is about an inch shorter),
and less than 1/4" thick. ALWAYS, NEW FREEDOM, and STAYFREE make
a basic ultrathin. KOTEX and SURE & NATURAL both make a "long"
ultrathin, about an inch longer. ALWAYS has a slender ultra-thin maxipad pad to prevent shifting. ALWAYS and STAYFREE have a long ultra-
thin with wings.

THIN MAXIPADS   These are the same overall size as the ultra-thin
pads but up to half an inch thick. ALWAYS are narrower in the middle,
with side channels to prevent overflow. ALWAYS SLENDER THIN are
narrower than most thin pads; KOTEX thin supers are thicker; NEW
FREEDOM THIN DEODORANT contain baking soda to neutralize odors.

REGULAR MAXIPADS   These are the most popular pads, account-
ing for 45 percent of all menstrual pad sales. A regular maxipad is
about the same size as the thin or ultrathin, but it can be up to three
fourths of an inch thick. Maxipads are available with baking powder
as a deodorant (ALWAYS, STAYFREE CLASSIC); slender (NATRACARE),
long (SURE & NATURAL), or hourglass shaped (KOTEX PROFILE); super
(KOTEX, NATRACARE, STAYFREE); and with wings and channels (AL-
WAYS MAXI WITH WINGS).

All are anchored with one or more adhesive strips. For tradition-
alists, one pad, KOTEX FEMININE NAPKINS, is still made with tabs to
fit an elastic belt.

EXTRA-PROTECTION PADS   These pads, such as ALWAYS CURVED,
KOTEX CURVED, and KOTEX CURVED SUPER, are U-shaped, with elastic gathers at the side that curve the pad up in front and back to cup
your body and prevent leaks. KOTEX SECURE HOLD, STAYFREE SURE

FIT regular and super, and ALWAYS long super all have wings. The AL-WAYS pad is contoured and has channels at the sides to prevent over-flow. The KOTEX pad curves. The STAYFREE is shaped higher in the center to meet your body, and has a 4-inch-long sponge in the middle.

MAXIMUM-PROTECTION PADS   These pads are too thick and bulky to be worn under clothes. They are meant to keep you and your bedclothes dry through nights of heavy flow. The first pad in this category was the 11" KOTEX OVERNITE, introduced in 1981, followed by NEW FREEDOM MAXIMUMS and STAYFREE SUPERLONG MAXI. ALWAYS OVERNIGHT WITH WINGS adds an extra touch of security.

TAMPONS

Like menstrual pads, tampons have a history that goes back several thousand years. Egyptian women used tampons made of papyrus. Roman women used soft wool; Indonesians, vegetable fiber; north Africans, roots and grass; Japanese, a paper tampon held in place with a kind of wraparound bandage called *kama* (meaning pony). The first commercial American tampon was invented by a Denver physician named Earle Haas who introduced his creation, TAMPAX, in 1936, and ran right into a barricade of prejudice, ignorance, and misinformation.

TAMPON MYTHS AND MISINFORMATION

Given the intimate nature of the tampon, it's not surprising how many myths there are about its use. The idea that you can lose your virginity to a tampon is only one of many old wives' tales.

MYTH 1: VIRGINS CAN'T USE TAMPONS.   The false assumption here is that an intact hymen (a membrane that stretches across the vaginal opening) covers the entrance entirely, thus preventing virgins from inserting a tampon. Not true. The hymen is anchored at the edges of the vaginal opening and extends toward the center, rather like a doughnut. It is rare to find a hymen without any opening in the center.

Given our individual differences, the hymeneal opening is larger in some women than in others, but it is almost always large enough to permit at least a limited internal gynecological examination, and definitely large enough to allow menstrual fluid to flow out. Any girl who has begun menstruating while still a virgin already has proof that she can use a tampon. A slim tampon such as TAMPAX JUNIOR is likely to be most comfortable at first. For days of heavier flow, the TAMPAX SLENDER or the JUNIOR backed up with a menstrual pad works well.

MYTH 2: WOMEN WHO USE TAMPONS AREN'T VIRGINS ANYMORE.

The assumption here is that inserting a tampon tears the hymen. Not true. Using a tampon may gently stretch the natural opening in the hymen, but it will not tear the tissue. What some women may interpret as deflowering via tampon is a twinge of pain caused by trying to force a tampon past dry labia and clenched muscles. Like other tissues, the vaginal mucous membranes may dry or moisten in response to tension. Like muscles elsewhere, the vaginal muscles tighten in anticipation of pain. When you are relaxed, the tissues become naturally moist and the muscles loosen. When inserting a tampon, practice helps. So does lubricating the tip of the tampon with a water-soluble lubricant such as K-Y JELLY. (Do not use petroleum jelly. It does not dissolve in water and is very hard to wash off.)

MYTH 3: WEARING A TAMPON IS SEXUALLY STIMULATING.

No way. If properly inserted, tampons do not touch the clitoris, and they touch the labia only in passing. Once properly in place in the vagina, they produce no sensation at all. In fact, using a tampon can be so comfortable that a woman may forget to remove it, only to be reminded by leakage of menstrual fluid from a saturated tampon.

MYTH 4: TAMPONS CAN GET LOST IN THE VAGINA OR FLOAT UP INTO THE ABDOMINAL CAVITY.

The first is unlikely; the second impossible. The only internal exit from the vagina is the cervix, the entrance through which sperm move into the uterus. This opening is simply too small to permit a tampon through. There is absolutely no way that a tampon can "float" upward from the vagina to the uterus or any other internal organ.

As for its getting lost in the vagina, well, if you snag the tampon string around the tampon when you insert it, you may have some slight difficulty in locating the string when it's time to remove the tampon. Or, if you have intercourse with a tampon in place (not a recommended procedure), the penis may push the string up or move the tampon to one side inside the vagina. The tampon isn't lost; it's just not where you expect it to be. If the string's the problem, just reach slightly higher until you find it. If the tampon has been pushed upward or sideways, try squatting to shorten the vaginal canal; then reach—gently—for the tampon. Don't panic if it takes a minute to find it. Unless your fingers are so short that they cannot stretch to the top of the vagina (and this is very rare), you will soon corral the tampon. Apocryphal stories about women rushing to the emergency room for tampon retrieval have less to do with lost tampons than with a woman's reluctance to touch her own body.

REAL TROUBLE, REAL FACTS

The original TAMPAX tampon, made of cotton rolled into a cylinder shape with a string attached for easy removal, offered many advantages over external pads, but it was not completely protective against leaks.

As fiber technology expanded after World War II, tampon manufacturers began to experiment with new materials, adding synthetic fibers to increase absorbency. They also began to play with design. Procter & Gamble's RELY was a revolutionary product, tiny sponges and super-absorbent synthetic fibers floating free inside a dense synthetic net, a package meant to absorb menstrual fluid and balloon up inside the vagina.

RELY went into test markets in 1974 and into general distribution six years later. It was very effective, with consumer word-of-mouth reports good enough to trigger an absorbency competition that soon produced *super* and *super-plus* tampons containing extraordinarily absorbent synthetic fibers such as carboxymethylcellulose, polyesters, and polyacrylate rayon. Tampons were so large that some women actually found it difficult to insert them unless heavy menstrual bleeding made the vaginal walls slick enough to allow the tampon in.

Up until the time RELY was introduced, through several thousand years of tampon history, there had never been a serious, documented claim of tampon-related injury. In the United States, 40 years' experience with tampons had been so uneventful, medically speaking, that the Food and Drug Administration rated tampons as Class II Medical Devices, a category defined as *safe and effective*. As a result, tampon manufacturers were not required to test new products as, for example, drug companies must test new drugs to be sure they work without injuring a patient.

Perhaps it was too good to last.

Within a year after RELY appeared on drugstore shelves, disturbing reports began to filter in about tampons in general and RELY in particular. The problem was two-fold: vaginal injury and vaginal infection.

VAGINAL INJURY   The first warning about the new, super-absorbent tampons was an increasing number of injuries to vaginal tissues. In 1980, a study from the Medical College of Wisconsin in Milwaukee turned up evidence that using tampons dried the vaginal tissues, causing "layering" (flaking) of the vaginal walls and micro-ulcerations, ulcers too small to be seen with the naked eye. These tiny injuries were found most often in women who were using super-absorbent tampons or using tampons all month long, even when they were not menstruating, to soak up the normal, lubricating vaginal secretions, which they considered offensive. Women who used regular-size tampons and used them only when menstruating were much less likely to develop these tissue changes. The tissue damage, however, seemed to be temporary; it disappeared when the women stopped using large tampons and restricted their use to the days of menstrual flow, which is current medical advice for any woman who uses tampons.

VAGINAL INFECTION   Toxic shock syndrome (TSS) is an infection caused by toxin from the bacteria called *Staphylococcus aureus*, which grows in the nose, throat, and vagina, as well as in wounds, including surgical wounds, and vaginal wounds after delivery. The infection, first diagnosed formally in 1978 among children, causes a high fever, vomiting, diarrhea, a sunburn-like rash, peeling skin on fingers and toes, liver or kidney failure, and a rapid drop in blood pressure leading to shock (a shutdown of body systems).

Staph organisms have always been with us, so it is likely that TSS has been around pretty much forever. What was new was the rapid increase in the number of cases and who got sick. The overwhelming majority of the cases diagnosed in the period immediately surrounding the introduction of the super tampons occurred among women who were using a super-absorbent tampon during menstrual bleeding. This high incidence of TSS among healthy young women of reproductive age was confirmed in a three-state study in 1981, and soon there were statistics to show that for women using the most absorbent tampons, the risk of TSS was 30 times higher than for women who did not use tampons; for women using the least absorbent tampons, the risk was 2 to 3 times higher than for nonusers. About 5 percent of all cases were fatal. Between 1984, when the government began tracking TSS, and 1989, there were 49 deaths.

Every brand of tampon then on the market was implicated in at least a few cases of TSS, but one brand—RELY—showed up more frequently than any other, perhaps because when Procter & Gamble mailed out 60 million samples of the new tampon in 1980, they reached 80 percent of the households in this country. Women wishing to use a more absorbent tampon had RELY right at hand—suggesting that part of its problem was the result of its sampling success.

Eventually, the TSS epidemic was traced to the use of super-absorbent materials, which provide a geometrically increased number of surfaces on which bacteria can multiply to produce TSST-1, the toxin that causes the disease. By 1981, when RELY and a number of other super-absorbency tampons were withdrawn from the market, tampon sales had fallen for all brands. Before the introduction of RELY, nearly three quarters of all women in the United States had used tampons on a regular basis. By 1981, that fraction had dropped to half.

TAMPON STANDARDS

When the super tampons disappeared, the incidence of TSS among menstruating women dropped sharply. To protect healthy women who chose to use tampons, the FDA ruled in 1982 that tampon packages must provide a list of TSS symptoms and the advice to choose the lowest absorbency possible.

But this advice was hard to follow, as there were no standard terms to define tampon absorbency. One company's super tampon may or may not have been more absorbent than another's regular or super-plus version, so women had no practical way to compare products.

For several years, the FDA discussed and debated and dithered about standards, bending first one way, then the other. A task force representing consumers, government, and manufacturers was set up and then disbanded in 1984 when they could not agree on ways to describe a tampon's absorbency. The FDA then proposed a rating system using the letters A through F. This scheme would allow manufacturers to use their own terms, as long as they also put one of the letters on the box; however, consumers, health professionals, and manufacturers alike called the plan confusing and inconsistent. Finally, in 1989, the FDA created a new proposal linking existing descriptive terms such as *junior, regular,* and *super* to specific amounts of liquid absorbed. As of March 1990, all tampons sold in the United States were required to conform to and carry copy describing this rating system, shown in the table below.

FDA TAMPON STANDARDS		
Flow	*Absorbency (grams of fluid)*	*Label Terms*
light	6 grams and less	junior
light to moderate	6 to 9 grams	regular
moderate to heavy	9 to 12 grams	super
heavy	12 to 15 grams	super plus

Standardizing tampon absorbency does not completely eliminate the risk of TSS. Although the incidence has declined dramatically, with only 54 cases in 1992, toxic shock syndrome in menstruating women has not disappeared. In 1995, statisticians estimate that as many as 1 to 17 of every 100,000 menstruating girls and women will contract TSS each year. It is common among women younger than 30 who are using tampons; women aged 15 to 19 have the highest risk. Overall, despite changes in tampon construction and size, the risk is still as much as 48 percent higher among tampon users.

This risk appears to be linked to materials still used in all the major brands of tampons. All have an absorbent core of cotton or rayon fiber. Some are treated with a surfactant or finishing agent such as a polysorbate that increases absorbency. The core is rolled or folded, covered with a fine-mesh fabric made of rayon or polyethylene/polyester, and anchored with a cotton cord for removing the tampon. The entire package is fitted into a cardboard or plastic applicator or simply wrapped in plastic without any applicator. The latter is called a digital tampon because it is inserted with the finger (digit).

In 1994, Philip M. Tierno Jr. and Bruce A. Hanna, of the department of microbiology and pathology at the New York University School of Medicine, published the results of a study in which they had inoculated tampons with *Staph aureus*. Their data shows that bacteria thrives on tampons containing rayon and polyester, producing large quantities of TSST-1, the toxin that causes toxic shock syndrome. But the microorganisms do not seem to fare well on two brands of all-cotton tampons (NATRACARE, TERRA FEMME) made without a mesh cover. At the end of the study, there were no detectable amounts of TSST-1 on these tampons.

Tierno and Hanna concluded that women using ordinary, rayon, or rayon and cotton tampons were at a higher risk of developing TSS. They called for other scientists to verify their findings of no toxin on the all-cotton tampons. They said it might be "prudent to suggest the exclusive use of all-cotton fibers" in tampons. In short, they seem to be recommending a return to the original, all-cotton tampon introduced as TAMPAX so many years ago.

CHOOSING AN EFFECTIVE TAMPON

Defining an effective tampon is easy. It is absorbent enough to protect against leaks for a reasonable amount of time, but not so absorbent that it dries the vaginal tissues. It is easy to insert, comfortable to wear, easy to remove, and a cinch to dispose of.

COMFORT AND CONVENIENCE Happiness for a menstruating woman may be a tampon that doesn't pinch going in or pull coming out. In part this depends on the applicator, which may be plastic or cardboard. The former usually feels smoother than the latter, but that may not be your only concern.

Cardboard is biodegradable; plastic isn't. Cardboard is flushable; plastic isn't. If you want a tampon with an applicator, the best of both worlds may be PLAYTEX ULTIMATES or TAMPAX SATIN TOUCH, which contain flushable cardboard applicators treated to feel as smooth as plastic. One interesting variation, KOTEX CURVED, has a curved applicator. It promises to go in easier and position the tampon better because it follows the natural curve of the vagina. NATRA-CARE and o.b., which do not have applicators, are a pleasure to pack in your purse and they satisfy environmental concerns, but may be slightly uncomfortable to insert on a light day when the vaginal tissues are relatively dry.*

Comfort also depends on using the right size tampon. If you are using a large tampon or a very absorbent one on a day when your flow is light, the surface of the tampon may not be completely satu-

---

* Tampons without applicators are not new inventions. In 1945, nine years after Tampax was introduced, there were at least four other applicatorless brands on the market: CASHAY, DALE, HOLLYPAX, and WIX. According to a contemporary marketing study from Fawcett Publications, 37 percent of all women using tampons in 1942 used homemade tampons, tampons without applicators.

rated, which means that it may tear at the vaginal walls when you pull it out, causing microscopic injuries.

All tampons except TAMPAX and the all-cotton SEVENTH GENERATION have a cotton cord attached at the bottom. When you pull on the cord to remove the tampon, you exert uneven pressure along the tampon, greater at the bottom, lighter at the top. As a result, the tampon may come out in a series of jerky movements. The cord on SEVENTH GENERATION and TAMPAX is stitched evenly up the center for the full length of the tampon. Pulling this string exerts even pressure all the way up the tampon, which should come out smoothly.

LEAK PROTECTION   Each month, a typical woman loses an average of 4 to 12 teaspoons of menstrual fluid or between 20 and 60 grams. The 1990 FDA absorbency guidelines, based on a tampon's ability to absorb specific amounts of fluid, go a long way toward enabling a consumer to choose a comfortable, protective product.

Clearly, a tampon's absorbency influences its ability to protect against leaks, but changing tampons as often as needed is also important. On days of heavy flow, even the most absorbent tampons will leak if allowed to become so saturated that they cannot cope with the sudden discharge that occurs when, for example, you stand up after you have been sitting for a while.

Your activity level can also affect a tampon's performance. For example, while you are bouncing around on the tennis court, your tampon is bouncing around inside you. One bounce may move the tampon just a bit and allow leakage. Many women find it provident to provide backup with a securely anchored menstrual pad, perhaps an ultra-thin maxi with wings.

Another important difference between one tampon and another when it comes to preventing leaks is the shape the tampon assumes as it expands inside the vagina. Drop a KOTEX SECURITY, SEVENTH GENERATION, NATRACARE, o.b., PLAYTEX, or TAMPAX tampon into a pot of water, and you will see that they are made differently and expand in different ways. KOTEX and TAMPAX tampons expand somewhat in length and width, but NATRACARE, o.b., PLAYTEX, and SEVENTH GENERATION expand primarily in width to end up looking like a small bell or even a barrel, wider overall than KOTEX or TAMPAX.

Logically, tampons that expand sideways should block leaks more efficiently, but in practice this may or may not be true. When rating tampons in 1995, *Consumer Reports* found that o.b. regular absorbed test fluid similar in thickness to menstrual fluid at a slower rate than

did KOTEX and PLAYTEX regulars, but faster than TAMPAX, while TAM-
PAX tampons consistently absorbed smaller amounts of saline (salt) solution than the other brands. The *Consumer Reports* survey did not
include the NATRACARE or SEVENTH GENERATION brands, but the
study on toxic shock syndrome from New York University Hospital
(see pages 48–49) showed cotton tampons equal in absorbency to
other tampons in the same category (regular, super, etc.).

DISPOSABILITY   Cotton and cotton/rayon tampons, rayon coverings,
and cotton or rayon strings are natural materials that degrade completely; synthetic (polyethylene/polyester) coverings do not. NATRA-
CARE and SEVENTH GENERATION tampons are entirely degradable.
Whether this influences your choice of tampon depends on how con-
cerned you are about environmental issues.

   For a table comparing a wide selection of different tampons on
the market see pages 52–56.

COMPARING THE PRODUCTS: TAMPONS

Tampon	Applicator	Composition	Comments
JUNIOR* **(ABSORBS UP TO 6 GRAMS LIQUID)**			
TAMPAX (Tambrands)	cardboard, flushable	cotton fiber, rayon wrap, cotton cord	expands lengthwise; cord stitched down length of entire tampon
REGULAR **(ABSORBS 6–9 GRAMS LIQUID)**			
KOTEX CURVED (Kimberly Clark)	plastic (curved), nonflushable	rayon fiber, rayon wrap, cotton cord	rolled cylinder, expands in width and length
KOTEX SECURITY (Kimberly Clark)	plastic, rounded, nonflushable	rayon fiber, rayon wrap, cotton cord	expands in width and length
KOTEX SECURITY SLENDER (Kimberly Clark)	plastic, rounded, nonflushable	rayon fiber, rayon wrap, cotton cord	expands in width and length
NATRACARE (Natracare)	no applicator	cotton, cotton cord	rolled layers expand sideways in a barrel shape
o.b. (Personal Products)	no applicator; tampon has rounded tip	rayon and cotton fibers, polyethylene/ polyester wrap, rayon or cotton cord	15 rolled layers expand in a bell shape; cord attached at bottom
o.b. applicator (Personal Products)	cardboard, flushable	rayon, cotton, polyethylene polyester cover	15 rolled layers expand in a bell shape; cord attached at bottom

* TAMPAX LITES, a subregular, junior-abosorbency tampon, was introduced in 1994.

Tampon	Applicator	Composition	Comments
PLAYTEX (Playtex)	plastic, nonflushable	rayon and cotton fibers, polypropylene cover, cotton cord	tampon expands in a tulip shape; wider at top than at bottom; cord attached at bottom; also contains polysorbate-20; deodorant version has fragrance; packed in plastic disposal pouch
PLAYTEX SILK GLIDE (Playtex)	flushable "SILKGLIDE" cardboard, rounded tip	rayon fiber, rayon polyethylene and polyester wrap, cotton cord	see PLAYTEX (above); scented version contains fragrance
PLAYTEX SOFT COMFORT (Playtex)	plastic, nonflushable	rayon, cotton string, may contain cotton fiber	see PLAYTEX (above)
SEVENTH GENERATION (Seventh Generation)	cardboard, flushable	cotton, paper wrap, cotton cord	expands sideways; chlorine-free; cord stitched length of tampon
TAMPAX COMPAK (Tambrands)	plastic, nonflushable; half the length of a normal tampon in packet; when opened, telescoping applicator expands to full size	rayon fiber, rayon wrap, cotton cord	expands lengthwise; cord stitched down length of entire tampon
TAMPAX NATURAL (Tambrands)	cardboard, flushable	cotton with cotton overwrap	expands lengthwise; cord stitched down length of entire tampon

Tampon	Applicator	Composition	Comments
TAMPAX ORIGINAL (Tambrands)	cardboard, flushable	cotton fiber, rayon wrap, cotton cord	expands lengthwise; cord stiched down length of entire tampon
TAMPAX PLASTIC (Tambrands)	plastic, nonflushable	rayon fiber, rayon wrap, cotton cord	expands lengthwise; cord stitched down length of entire tampon
TAMPAX SATIN TOUCH (Tambrands)	flushable "SATIN BOARD" (cardboard, rounded tip)	rayon fiber, rayon wrap, cotton cord	expands lengthwise; cord stitched down length of entire tampon
TAMPAX SLENDER (Tambrands)	cardboard, flushable	rayon fiber, rayon wrap, cotton cord	expands lengthwise; cord stitched down length of entire tampon
TERRA FEMME (Bio Business International)	no applicator	cotton, cotton cord	chlorine-free
SUPER (ABSORBS 9–12 GRAMS LIQUID)			
KOTEX CURVED (Kimberly Clark)	plastic (curved), nonflushable	rayon fiber, rayon wrap, cotton cord	rolled cylinder, expands in width and length
KOTEX SECURITY (Kimberly Clark)	plastic, rounded, nonflushable	rayon fiber, rayon wrap, cotton cord	expands in width and length
NATRACARE (Natracare)	no applicator	cotton, cotton cord	rolled layers expand sideways in a barrel shape
o.b. (Personal Products)	no applicator; tampon has rounded tip	rayon and cotton fibers, polyethylene/ polyester wrap, rayon or cotton cord	15 rolled layers expand in a bell shape; cord attached at bottom

Tampon	Applicator	Composition	Comments
o.b. applicator (Personal Products)	cardboard, flushable	rayon, cotton, polyethylene polyester cover	15 rolled layers expand in a bell shape; cord attached at bottom
PLAYTEX (Playtex)	plastic, nonflushable	rayon and cotton fiber, polypropylene cover, cotton cord	tampon expands in a tulip shape; wider at top than at botton; cord attached at bottom; also contains polysorbate-20; deodorant version has fragrance; packed in plastic disposal pouch
PLAYTEX SOFT COMFORT (Playtex)	plastic, non-flushable	rayon, cotton cord, may contain cotton fiber	see PLAYTEX (above)
TAMPAX (Tambrands)	cardboard, flushable	rayon and coton fibers, rayon wrap, cotton cord	expands lengthwise; cord stitched down length of entire tampon
TAMPAX COMPAK (Tambrands)	plastic, nonflushable; half the length of a normal tampon in packet; when opened, telescoping applicator expands to full size	rayon fiber, rayon wrap, cotton cord	expands lengthwise; cord stitched down length of entire tampon
TERRA FEMME (Bio Business International)	no applicator	cotton, cotton cord	chlorine-free

Tampon	Applicator	Composition	Comments
SUPER PLUS (ABSORBS 12–15 GRAMS LIQUID)			
KOTEX SECURITY (Kimberly Clark)	plastic, rounded, nonflushable	rayon fiber, rayon wrap, cotton cord	expands in width and length
PLAYTEX (Playtex)	plastic, nonflushable	rayon and cotton fiber, polypropylene cover, cotton cord	tampon expands in a tulip shape; wider at top than at botton; cord attached at bottom; also contains polysorbate-20; deodorant version has fragrance; packed in plastic disposal pouch
TAMPAX (Tambrands)	cardboard, flushable	rayon fiber, rayon wrap, cotton cord	expands lengthwise; cord stitched down length of entire tampon

Sources: Products on sale in New York City, summer 1995. o.b. package insert, Personal Products Company. Promotional material from NATRACARE, SEVENTH GENERATION.

PREMENSTRUAL SYNDROME (PMS) AND MENSTRUAL CRAMPS

PMS is a collection of physical and psychological symptoms that start right after ovulation and end when menstrual bleeding begins. Menstrual cramps occur during the menstrual period; they have no connection to PMS.

PRESCRIPTION DRUGS FOR PMS

PMS symptoms such as breast tenderness, bloating, sleeplessness, and emotional ups and downs appear to be linked to rising and falling levels of the female sex hormones, estrogen and progesterone. Right after ovulation, estrogen levels fall and progesterone levels rise; the situation is reversed when menstrual bleeding begins.

Some doctors prescribe progesterone, as a suppository or pill, for relief of these symptoms, but no controlled study has ever turned up evidence that women with low levels of progesterone are at higher risk of PMS. An alternative is oral contraceptives to block ovulation and maintain even hormonal levels, but here, too, there is an absence of scientific proof to show the treatment works. In very severe cases of PMS, there is the possibility of pushing a woman into false menopause by prescribing LUPRON or SYNAREL, synthetic versions of gonadotropin-releasing agonists, natural hormones in the body that block the production of female sex hormones. This is complicated and tricky therapy that requires a patient to take small amounts of female sex hormones to prevent an increased risk of osteoporosis and other menopausal effects. It is also very expensive; a treatment of truly last resort.

In 1995, a study directed by Mier Steiner at St. Joseph's Hospital in Hamilton, Ontario, involving several hundred women at seven Canadian clinics, randomly assigned women with severe PMS to one of two groups, the first given the antidepressant fluoxetine (PROZAC); the second, a placebo. Half the women given PROZAC reported at least a moderate reduction in symptoms as compared with only one quarter of the women getting a placebo. Although many women use antidepressants to relieve anxiety associated with PMS, as well as to alleviate problems caused by insomnia, this is the first study specifically directed at the use of antidepressants to relieve PMS.

NONPRESCRIPTION DRUGS
FOR PMS AND MENSTRUAL CRAMPS

If your premenstrual days are only mildly uncomfortable and you have menstrual cramps only once in a while, your symptoms will almost certainly be soothed by a simple analgesic or one of the relatively mild combination menstrual products available without prescription. Check the labels, and you will find that all combination products conform to one of two basic formulas, either a diuretic or a diuretic plus analgesic.

ANALGESICS   The uterus is a muscle that, like all muscles, contracts and relaxes. During menstruation, the contractions become stronger owing to the production of *prostaglandins,* natural substances made by cells in the wall of the uterus. The simplest remedy for menstrual cramps is an OTC analgesic. Plain aspirin (ANACIN, ASCRIPTIN, BAYER, BUFFERIN, ECOTRIN), ibuprofen (ADVIL, MOTRIN-IB, NUPRIN, PAMPRIN-IB), and naproxen (ALEVE) are likely to be the most effective because they are *prostaglandin inhibitors,* substances that reduce the effects of prostaglandins and inhibit the formation of clots and thus relieve painful uterine contractions caused by the passage of large clots through the uterine cervix into the vaginal canal. However, all three analgesics may irritate the lining of the stomach, sometimes seriously enough to make it bleed.

The analgesic in most combination menstrual products is acetaminophen (MIDOL PMS, MIDOL MAXIMUM STRENGTH MENSTRUAL FORMULA, PAMPRIN, PREMSYN PMS), which relieves pain without irritating the stomach but is not a prostaglandin inhibitor. DIUREX contains potassium salicylate and salicylamide, which are related to aspirin.

DIURETICS   The FDA classifies ammonium chloride, caffeine, and pamabrom (a derivative of theophylline, a drug used to treat asthma) as safe and effective diuretics to relieve water retention and bloating right before and during your period. If you customarily drink coffee, tea, or colas, however, the caffeine in these products will add to your daily total and may make you feel jumpy or interfere with your sleep.

SEDATIVES   Pyrilamine maleate, an antihistamine used in some combination cold and allergy products such as POLYHISTINE and TRIAMINIC, is included in some combination menstrual products. It makes some people drowsy.

COMPARING THE PRODUCTS:
SELECTED OTC REMEDIES FOR
PMS AND MENSTRUAL DISCOMFORT

Product	Analgesic(s)	Diuretic	Sedative
AQUA BAN (Thompson Medical)	—	pamabrom (50 mg)	—
DIUREX LONG ACTING (Alva-Amco Pharmacal Companies)	acetaminophen, potassium salicylate	caffeine	—
MIDOL MAXIMUM STRENGTH (Sterling Health)	acetaminophen (500 mg)	caffeine (60 mg)	pyrilamine maleate (15 mg)
MIDOL PMS (Sterling Health)	acetaminophen (500 mg)	pamabrom (25 mg)	pyrilamine maleate (15 mg)
PAMPRIN (Chattem)	acetaminophen (250 mg), magnesium salicylate (250 mg)	pamabrom (25 mg)	—
PREMSYN PMS (Chattem)	acetaminophen (500 mg)	pamabrom (25 mg)	pyrilamine maleate (15 mg)

Sources: Products on sale in New York City, summer 1995.

HERBAL REMEDIES

Herbal medicine has a long and honored history, particularly in relation to menstrual pain. American pioneer women used elder bark tea for cramps; Native Americans used wild ginger; Central and South American women, cypress.

Today, herbal products enjoy a burgeoning popularity, especially among those of us who want to live "naturally," avoiding all "chemical" drugs. The problem, of course, is that all substances with medical effects, including herbal substances, are chemicals. Any herbal product strong enough to alleviate cramps or relieve premenstrual discomfort demands to be treated with a certain respect. Never take an herbal medication casually just because it comes without prescription.

The following table comments on a selection of herbs used for relief of menstrual discomfort.

HERBS USED TO
RELIEVE MENSTRUAL DISCOMFORT

Herbal tea brewed from	Function	Comments
Buchu Leaves	mild diuretic	safe for healthy people; effectiveness not proven
Chamomile	antispasmodic	safe and effective for healthy people; may cause allergic reactions in sensitive individuals
Dandelion	mild diuretic (leaves), mild laxative (roots)	safe for healthy people; effectiveness not proven
Ginger	antinausea effect	safe and effective in normal doses for healthy people; very large doses may depress the central nervous system
Ginseng Root	relieves general discomfort	contains small amounts of phytoestrogens (estrogen-like compounds in plants); may cause painful breast swelling; safety and effectiveness not proven
Nettle	diuretic	safe and effective for healthy people
Parsley	mild diuretic	safe for healthy people; effectiveness not proven
Uva Ursi	diuretic	safe and effective for healthy people

Sources: James A. Duke, *Handbook of Medicinal Herbs* (Boca Raton, FL: CRC Press, 1988). Varro E. Tyler, *Hoosier Home Remedies* (West Lafayette, IN: Purdue University Press, 1985). Varro E. Tyler, *The New Honest Herbal* (Philadelphia, PA: George F. Stickley, 1987).

SOURCES

"Always category SKU organizer chart" and additional correspondence, Proctor & Gamble, February 1995.

Dickinson, Robert Latou, "Tampons as menstrual guards," *Journal of the American Medical Association*, June 16, 1945.

Duke, James A., *Handbook of Medicinal Herbs* (Boca Raton, FL: CRC Press, 1988).

"Dysmenorrhea," The American College of Obstetricians and Gynecologists, March 1991.

Gossel, Thomas A., "Tampon absorbency and the risk of toxic shock syndrome," *U.S. Pharmacist,* November 1990.

"Kimberly-Clark introduces curved tampon," press release, Kimberly-Clark, March 16, 1994.

The Merck Manual, 16th ed. (Rahway, NJ: Merck Research Laboratories, 1992).

"New tampon regulations," *FDA Drug Bulletin,* April 1990.

"OTC pain relief primer," *FDA Consumer,* January-February 1995.

Papazian, Ruth, "Pain, pain, go away," *FDA Consumer,* Jan.-Feb. 1995.

"Study finds Prozac can relieve severe PMS," *New York Times,* June 8, 1995.

"Tampon industry in throes of change after toxic shock," *Wall Street Journal,* February 26, 1981.

"Tampons and pads, should you use what Mom used?" *Consumer Reports,* January 1995.

Tierno, Philip M. Jr., and Bruce A. Hanna, "Propensity of tampons and barrier contraceptives to amplify *Staphylococcus aureus* toxic shock syndrome-1," *Infectious Diseases in Obstetrics and Gynecology,* 1994.

"Two Kansas women sue tampon makers Playtex, Tambrands," *Wall Street Journal,* May 31, 1994.

Tyler, Varro E., *Hoosier Home Remedies* (West Lafayette, IN: Purdue University Press, 1985).

——, *The New Honest Herbal* (Philadelphia, PA: George F. Stickley, 1987).

"Women at risk . . . dioxin and rayon in tampons" (1995) and additional press and promotional materials, Natracare, Inc.

CHAPTER 3

BIRTH CONTROL

There is no right more important than the right to control your reproductive life. The availability of safe, effective contraception is not a
luxury. It is a necessity. Anything that reduces our choice of birth control methods or interferes with our obtaining reproductive services
lessens our ability to participate fully in the social, economic, and political life of our society. Regardless of the method we choose, each of
us has the absolute right to adequate, unbiased information and full
availability of birth control.

Nothing illustrates the dilemma we face in balancing reproductive rights and risks better than the birth control pill.

THE PILL

It began as a gleam in Margaret Sanger's eye. The iron-willed founder
of Planned Parenthood wanted a cheap, safe, effective, chemical contraceptive for women. In fact, she said, the very future of the world
might depend on it.

Sanger was not alone in her quest. In Shrewsbury, Massachusetts, Gregory Goodman Pincus, the scientific director of the Worces-
ter Foundation for Experimental Biology and a consultant to G. D.
Searle, and his associate Min Chueh Chang were looking for a hormone that would prevent pregnancy. Practically next door, in Brook-
line, John Rock, M.D., of the Reproductive Study Center, was looking
for a hormone to "cure" infertility.

Knowing that estrogen caused cancer of the breast and uterus in
laboratory animals, the two groups had, independent of each other,
settled on the second female hormone, progesterone. In 1952, a year
after Sanger gave Pincus a check for $2,100 as a down payment on
one year's research toward a birth control pill, Pincus and Rock began
working together, using natural progesterone obtained from pregnant

sows. But the hormone was scarce, expensive, and ineffective except in extraordinarily large doses. The creation of synthetic progesterone-like compounds in the early 1950s offered an acceptable alternative, and in 1956, Pincus, Chang, and Rock handed Sanger her prize: a progestin-only birth control pill made with G. D. Searle's norethynodrel.*

The new progestin pill seemed to be the perfect reversible contraceptive. It inhibited ovulation, but once a woman stopped taking it, she began ovulating again and could become pregnant. But it had been tested on fewer than a hundred women—medical students, patients at Rock's fertility clinic, and "volunteers" in local mental hospitals—so it was impossible to be sure the results were valid. What Pincus and Rock needed was a place to run a larger trial.

They picked Puerto Rico, in part because it had a large population of women of childbearing age; in part, to avoid legal problems. At the time, Americans held decidedly mixed views of contraception. In some states, such as New York, birth control was generally available. In others, such as Massachusetts, the law threatened five years' in jail or $1,000 in fines for anyone selling contraception. As journalist Paul Vaughn noted in his 1970 history *The Pill on Trial,* Puerto Rico had the "advantage of being safely out of sight of the bluenose brigade."

During the trials, the researchers discovered that the compound they were testing contained traces of estrogen substances. When they tried to "purify" it, women taking the pill developed breakthrough bleeding (spotting between menstrual periods), and there was concern that it might not protect them against pregnancy. Pincus and Rock put the estrogen back, creating a "combination" pill with 10 mg (milligrams) progestin and 150 mcg (micrograms; a microgram is 1/1000 of a milligram) estrogen, nearly five times the amount of estrogen in a modern "low dose" pill. On May 9, 1960, the Food and Drug Administration granted G. D. Searle permission to market the new combination pill, Enovid.

For a while all the news was good. The FDA said the pill was safe. Family planning experts, including Planned Parenthood's Alan Guttmacher, praised a "record of effectiveness no other contraceptive had matched." *Newsweek* reported Pincus's claim that the pill might protect against reproductive cancers. And women welcomed it. In 1961, nearly one million American women filled a first prescription

---

* "Progestins" is the collective term for natural progesterone and synthetic progesterone-like compounds.

for the new no-muss, no-fuss $3.50 oral contraceptive, moving it ahead of condoms, diaphragms, creams, and jellies to become the most popular form of reversible contraception.

"Before the pill, things were so complicated," says one medical writer, a member of the National Women's Health Network. "We were busy running careers, and every women I met at the time thought, anything is worth it. It was an immense convenience."

But soon there were problems. Within months after the pill went on sale, two California women died of pill-related blood clots. By the end of the year, G. D. Searle had reports of 132 cases of embolisms and 11 deaths among pill users. The FDA ordered the company to notify every doctor in the United States that taking birth control pills increased a woman's risk of blood clots. Then, in 1963, a U.S. Senate investigation discovered that the researchers had misrepresented the results of the pill trials.

The pill researchers had alluded to "thousands of women" and "47 patient years" of evidence from Puerto Rico to prove their contraceptive was safe and effective. In fact, only about 130 women had stuck with the pill for as long as a year. Another 90 or so had drifted in and out of the trial, taking the pill for periods ranging from one to nine months. According to Edris Rice-Wray, the physician who set up the Puerto Rico trials, the "47 patient years" represented the total number of months the pill was used by women who took it for more than two months, divided by 12. As for safety, no one had told the FDA that one fifth of the women who took the pill reported side effects such as headaches, dizziness, and stomach upset, some serious enough to make them leave the trial.

For several years, stories about unpleasant side effects continued to circulate among pill users, whose doctors often pooh-poohed their concerns. Then a self-described "sleep deprived mother of three" upset the applecart. Medical writer Barbara Seaman was completing an advanced science-writing fellowship at Columbia University in April 1968 when her professor insisted it would be "immoral" not to follow up on anecdotes about pill problems. Seaman took up the challenge, and one year later, in 1969, she published *The Doctors' Case Against the Pill,* a meticulously detailed account of what had gone wrong in creating, testing, and prescribing oral contraceptives. Drug companies called her book "unbalanced" and "unscientific," but Seaman stood her ground. "I knew how to read a medical journal," she says.

A copy of Seaman's book made its way to U.S. Senator Gaylord Nelson, chair of the Senate Subcommittee on Monopoly of the Select

Committee on Small Business, and Seaman was invited to work with Nelson's staff in preparing full-scale hearings on the pill. The hearings opened on January 14, 1970. For two months there was a steady stream of bad news about the pill. By March, when the Nelson hearings ended, pill use among American women had fallen 18 percent, and a newly energized cadre of female health activists had a promise from Secretary of Health, Education, and Welfare Robert Finch that the FDA would put a "patient product insert" into every package of oral contraceptives. In April, when the FDA seemed about to bow to pressure from doctors and pharmaceutical companies not to require the package inserts, a group of Washington, D.C. women set up camp outside the Secretary's office, chanting "The doctors gave the pill; the mothers, they got ill." That summer, the package inserts went into every container of birth control pills.

By now, the pill's more serious side effects had been traced to high doses of estrogen, particularly pills containing 0.05 mg (50 mcg) or more, the dose more than half the 8.5 million American pill users were getting. In 1969, the British Committee on Safety of Drugs recommended banning these high-dose pills. Although the FDA did not go along with the recommendation until 1988, prescriptions for high-estrogen pills declined steadily during the 1970s. As a result, the incidence of serious side effects went down and, for a while, so did the decibel level in arguments about the pill's safety. There was a short, sharp spike in 1975 when a report from the University of Colorado School of Medicine showed an increased risk of endometrial cancer among pill users, but the culprit was a particular form of birth control pills known as "sequentials" (21 estrogen-only pills followed by 7 progestin-only pills). When the FDA ordered the sequentials off the market, the cancer scare died down.

But it flared with a vengeance in 1981 when University of Southern California epidemiologists released the first of two reports showing an increased incidence of early (prior to age 40) breast cancer among women taking birth control pills for four years before a first full-term pregnancy or before age 25. Pill advocates cited the large Cancer and Steroid Hormone Study (CASH), which showed no increase in the risk of breast cancer among pill users. In 1989, however, the long-running Nurses Health Study in Boston showed the risk for "current users" to be 60 percent higher than that for nonusers. A subsequent reexamination of CASH showed a clear increase in risk for young women. In 1994, a Fred Hutchinson Cancer Research Center (Seattle) review of previous reviews and studies confirmed the link between early pill use and the early onset of breast cancer. In 1995, Louise A. Brinton and a team of researchers from the National Cancer Institute published a study of 2,203 breast cancer patients and 2,009 healthy women showing that women younger than 35 who had used birth control pills for six months or longer had a risk of breast cancer nearly twice that of women who had never used the pill.

At the same time, numerous studies continued to show that, as Gregory Goodman Pincus had predicted in 1961, taking combination birth control pills lowers the risk of ovarian and endometrial cancer, though a 1991 study from Canada provided ammunition for those who believed that taking the pill increases a woman's risk of cancer of the cervix.

Three years earlier, molecular biologists Mary M. Pater and Alan Pater and a group of colleagues at the Memorial University of New-foundland in St. John's had shown that inserting genetic material from herpes viruses that cause genital warts into rat cells and exposing the cells to progesterone turned the cells to cancer. They moved on to human cervical cells, inserting DNA from herpes viruses and bathing the cells in either the synthetic hormone dexamethasone or progester-one. Once again, the cells began to change, increasing their production of cancer-causing proteins that shut down the cell's normal tumor sup-presser genes, the genes that prevent the wild cell growth we call can-cer. One drug, however, seemed to block this process, at least in a test tube. The drug? RU-486, the "abortion pill" widely available in Europe and recently moved toward FDA approval in the United States.

Today, the birth control pill remains America's most popular method of reversible contraception. According to the 1993 Ortho Contraceptive Study from Ortho Pharmaceuticals, the nation's leading manufacturer of contraceptive products, 27 percent of the 67 million American women of reproductive age (15 to 50) have opted for per-manent birth control (sterilization); 25 percent use birth control pills; 7 percent rely on withdrawal or the rhythm method; 2 percent use a diaphragm. The FDA, which once warned against giving the pill to older women, now recommends it for the 10 million healthy non-smoking women over 40 who still need birth control.

In addition, many doctors prescribe the pill for a variety of non-contraceptive purposes, called "off-label" because they have not been formally approved by the FDA. "Oral contraceptives stabilize irregular periods," says Johanna F. Perlmutter, obstetrician and gynecologist at Beth Israel Hospital in Boston and assistant professor of obstetrics, gynecology, and reproductive medicine at Harvard Medical School.

"This is particularly important for young women who haven't yet established regular cycles; for women who do not ovulate on a regular basis and may be at risk for endometrial cancer; and for disease-free women, with irregular bleeding in the middle of the month, especially older women who might otherwise face surgical procedures to investigate what seems to be abnormal bleeding but is really a pattern leading to menopause."

If the pill is reliable contraception, it is definitely not a method of safe sex. "We are really clear that condoms are an essential way of protecting health, which means protecting against unintended pregnancy *and* sexually transmitted diseases," says Peggy Clarke, president of the American Social Health Association. "If you are sexually active, you need to think about condoms plus the pill."

Condoms are sold over-the-counter. Should pills be, too? That question is currently on the table at the FDA. In a 1994 survey by the American College of Obstetricians and Gynecologists, 86 percent of all respondents said no, arguing that women taking birth control pills should be monitored by their doctors. Among pill users, 91 percent said no. Selling the pill OTC may also be prejudicial to poor women who get their preventive health care and screening only through publicly subsidized family planning clinics. If we no longer require prescriptions for oral contraceptives, there will be a smaller market for these clinics, which may begin to shut down, depriving numbers of low-income women of health care.

Thirty-five years after it was introduced, the birth control pill still stirs debate. It frees women to control their reproductive lives but changes the environment of the reproductive tract to increase susceptibility to many sexually transmitted diseases. It raises a young woman's risk of breast cancer but lowers the risk of ovarian and endometrial cancer in women of all ages. It puts some women at risk of vascular and liver disease while protecting others from unnecessary surgery.

It is the best of pills, it is the worst of pills. And as Margaret Sanger predicted, it has changed the world forever.

SHOULD YOU TAKE THE PILL?

If you smoke; have a history of blood clots, heart disease, or high blood pressure; or have migraine headaches or undiagnosed vaginal bleeding or breast cancer; or have intercourse infrequently and do not need to use a contraceptive every day, your decision is simplicity itself: the pill is not for you.

On the other hand, if you do not smoke, if you are in good health, and if you have frequent intercourse, you may be a good candidate for the pill.

If you are over 35, your choice may be complicated by a debate between the FDA (which approves the use of drugs) and women's activists. Testifying in 1989 before the hearing about making the pill allowable for older women, Adriane Fugh-Berman, M.D., spokesperson for the National Women's Health Network, argued against raising the age limit. "Permitting older women to stay on the pill will increase long-term exposure," she said. "Known or suspected breast cancer is an absolute contraindication, and the incidence of breast cancer is higher in women older than 35. Since routine yearly mammography is recommended only after 50, women between 35 and 50 may be exposed to the pill while they have very small tumors that would be promoted by the pill. Pill users also have an additional risk of gallstones and liver disease, again higher among older women."

COMPARE THE RISKS AND BENEFITS

Below is a list of the proven and suspected side effects some women have suffered while using birth control pills.

- growth of uterine fibroids

- increased risk of breast cancer in young women

- increased risk of heart disease in older women

- change in menstrual patterns (spotting at midcycle)

- increased risk of vaginal yeast infection

- increased risk of migraines

- enlarged or tender breasts

- possible infertility after discontinuing the pill

- weight gain

- fluid retention that causes swollen breasts, wrists, ankles, and eyeballs*

---

* This is why some women find it uncomfortable to wear contact lenses while taking the pill.

- vaginal secretions

- increased risk of ectopic pregnancy

- acne; oily skin

- growth of body hair

- loss of hair

- bleeding between periods

This is not a catalog of random horrors. Most of these side effects are associated with the estrogens (ethinyl estradiol and mestranol) in oral contraceptives. A few, such as skin problems and weight gain, are linked to the progestins (ethynodiol diacetate, levonorgestrel, norethindrone, and norgestrel). Two new progestins—norgestimate and desogestrel—appear to be less likely to cause these problems. Women using oral contraceptives may find themselves at risk of skin pigmentation when exposed to sunlight, an effect that appears to be linked to the estrogens in the product. Sunscreen is a good idea, and at least one cosmetic company, Neutrogena, has run ads for pharmacists specifically suggesting that they offer their customers NEUTROGENA MOISTURE SPF 15 when they are on the pill.

Of course, the pill does have a positive side. According to the American College of Obstetricians and Gynecologists, oral contraceptives

- produce more regular menstrual cycles

- restore menstruation in women who do not ovulate

- reduce the incidence and severity of menstrual pain (dysmenorrhea)

- prevent or reduce the incidence of benign breast disease (fibrous tumors and cysts)

- prevent or reduce the incidence of pelvic inflammatory disease and ectopic pregnancy

- prevent or reduce the incidence of ovarian cysts (may not be true of low-estrogen pills)

- reduce the incidence of ovarian cancer and cancer of the endometrium (lining of the uterus)

COMPARE THE PRODUCTS

The pill is not one pill. It is several different kinds of pills, each with advantages and disadvantages.

MODERATE-DOSE PILLS   Until 1988, oral contraceptives contained as much as 100 mcg or more of estrogen, a "high dose" believed responsible for many of the serious side effects of the original birth control pills. In 1988, the FDA asked manufacturers of pills containing 75 to 100 mcg of estrogen to cease the manufacture and sale of these products because they were not more effective than lower-dose pills and appeared to be connected with a much higher rate of blood clotting disorders (stroke).

Today, the highest dose approved for contraceptive use is 50 mcg, an amount called "moderate." Moderate-dose pills (DEMULEN 1/50, NORINYL 1+50, ORTHO-NOVUM 1/50, OVRAL) are likely to produce estrogen-related side effects but are the most effective in preventing pregnancy. Of 100 women who use these pills for one year, fewer than one will become pregnant.* These pills are taken in a 21- or 28-day cycle.† If you miss one pill, taking two the next day may protect you, but check with your doctor to be sure.

LOW-DOSE COMBINATION PILLS   Low-dose combination pills (BREVICON, DEMULEN 1/35, LEVLEN, LOESTRIN 1.5/30 and 1/20, LO/OVRAL, MODICON, NORDETTE, NORINYL 1+35, ORTHO-CEPT, ORTHO-CYCLEN, ORTHO-NOVUM 1/35, ORTHOTRI-CYCLEN, OVCON 35, OVRETTE, TRI-LEVLEN, TRI-NORINYL) also contain a progestin plus estrogen, but the amount of estrogen is reduced to less than 40 mcg, and usually less than 35 mcg.

Several low-dose pills, such as ORTHO-NOVUM 7/7/7 and TRI-PHASIL, are *phasic* products, with three different combinations to be taken at different points in the menstrual cycle. Like moderate-dose pills, low-dose pills are packed either 21 or 28 to a container.

---

* This is a statistical average that permits us to express the failure rate (how many women become pregnant) in numbers smaller than one. For example, if these 100 women take birth control pills for two years and only one becomes pregnant, the failure rate per year is "less than one."

† Packages of 21 pills contain 21 hormone tablets. Packages of 28 pills contain 21 hormone tablets, plus 7 containing inert ingredients which are included so that you take one pill every day of the cycle.

Low-dose pills are slightly less effective than moderate-dose pills at preventing pregnancy. If 100 women use low-dose pills for one year, fewer than two will become pregnant. While this is still very low, it is twice the failure rate expected with moderate-dose pills. On the other hand, there seem to be fewer estrogen-related side effects associated with low-dose pills (less risk of blood clots, high blood pressure) but more progestin-related problems (acne, oily skin). If you miss one day, your best bet is to use additional protection (diaphragm, spermicide, condom) for the rest of your cycle.

MINI-PILLS   Mini-pills (MICRONOR, NOR QD, OVRETTE) contain a progestin but no estrogen, the formula for the original birth control pill created by Pincus, Rock, and Chang. Progestin-only pills produce progestin-related side effects such as skin problems, growth of body hair and thinning of scalp hair, and breakthrough bleeding. Of all the oral contraceptives, the progestin-only pill is the least effective at preventing pregnancy. If 100 women use this pill for one year, two or three may become pregnant. If you miss one day with the mini-pill, doubling up the next day will not work. You must use alternative contraception along with the pill for the rest of the menstrual cycle.

The table on the next three pages contains a detailed breakdown of the amounts of estrogen and progestin in several birth-control pills on the market.

COMPARING THE PRODUCTS: WHAT'S IN ORAL CONTRACEPTIVES?

Product (Supplier)	Estrogen	Progestin
BREVICON (Syntex)	35 mcg* ethinyl estradiol	0.50 mg norethindrone
DEMULEN 1/35 (G. D. Searle)	35 mcg ethinyl estradiol	1 mg ethynodiol diacetate
DEMULEN 1/50 (G. D. Searle)	50 mcg ethinyl estradiol	1 mg ethynodiol diacetate
LEVLEN (Berlex)	30 mcg ethinyl estradiol	0.15 mg levonorgestrel
LEVORA 0.15/30 (Hamilton Pharma)	30 mcg ethinyl estradiol	0.15 mg levonorgestrel
LOESTRIN 1/20† (Parke-Davis)	30 mcg ethinyl estradiol	1 mg norethindrone acetate
LOESTRIN 1.5/30† (Parke-Davis)	20 mcg ethinyl estradiol	1.50 mg norethindrone acetate
LO/OVRAL (Wyeth-Ayerst)	30 mcg ethinyl estradiol	0.30 mg norgestrel
MICRONOR (Ortho)	—	0.35 mg norethindrone
MODICON (Ortho)	35 mcg ethinyl estradiol	0.50 mg norethindrone
NORDETTE (Wyeth-Ayerst)	30 mcg ethinyl estradiol	0.15 mg levonorgestrel
NORINYL 1+35 (Syntex)	35 mcg ethinyl estradiol	1 mg norethindrone
NORINYL 1+50 (Syntex)	50 mcg mestranol	1 mg norethindrone
NOR QD (Syntex)	—	0.35 mg norethindrone

* A microgram (mcg) is 1/1000th of a milligram (mg)

† This product also comes with iron, shown by the symbol "FE," i.e., LOESTRIN FE.

Product (Supplier)	Estrogen	Progestin
ORTHO-CEPT (Ortho)	30 mcg ethinyl estradiol	0.15 mg desogestrel
ORTHO-CYCLEN (Ortho)	35 mcg ethinyl estradiol	0.25 mg norgestimate
ORTHO-NOVUM 1/35 (Ortho)	35 mcg ethinyl estradiol	1 mg norethindrone
ORTHO-NOVUM 1/50 (Ortho)	50 mcg mestranol	1 mg norethindrone
ORTHO-NOVUM[+] 7/7/7 (Ortho)	35 mcg, 35 mcg, 35 mcg ethinyl estradiol	0.50 mg, 0.75 mg, 1 mg norethindrone
ORTHO-NOVUM 10/11 (Ortho)	35 mcg ethinyl estradiol	0.50 mg norethindrone
ORTHO TRI-CYCLEN (Ortho)	35 mcg, 35 mcg, 35 mcg ethinyl estradiol[+]	0.180 mg, 0.215 mg, 0.250 mg norethindrone
OVCON 35 (Mead Johnson)	35 mcg ethinyl estradiol	0.40 mg norethindrone
OVCON 50 (Mead Johnson)	50 mcg ethinyl estradiol	1 mg norethindrone
OVRAL (Wyeth- Ayerst)	50 mcg ethinyl estradiol	0.50 mg norgestral
OVRETTE (Wyeth- Ayerst)	—	0.075 mg norgestrel
TRI-LEVLEN (Berlex)	30 mcg, 40 mcg, 30 mcg ethinyl estradiol	0.05 mg, 0.075 mg, 0.125 mg levonorgestrel
TRI-NORINYL[+] (Syntex)	35 mcg, 35 mcg, 35 mcg ethinyl estradiol	0.50 mg, 1.00 mg, 0.50 mg norethindrone
TRIPHASIL[+] (Wyeth-Ayerst)	30 mcg, 40 mcg, 30 mcg ethinyl estradiol	0.05 mg, 0.04 mg, 0.125 mg levonorgestrel

+ This is a three-phase product with 21 pills. The 28-day version contains an additional pill with inert (inactive) ingredients.

Product (Supplier)	Estrogen	Progestin
ZOVIA 1/30 (Watson)	35 mcg ethinyl estradiol	1 mg ethynodiol diacetate
ZOVIA 1/50 (Watson)	50 mcg ethinyl estradiol	1 mg ethynodiol diacetate

Note: Many oral contraceptives come in 21- and 28-day versions. The 21-day products have 21 pills with contraceptive ingredients; 28-day products have 21 pills with the same contraceptive ingredients plus 7 pills with inert ingredients.

Sources: Physicians' Desk Reference, 48th ed. (Montvale, NJ: Medical Economics Data, 1994). Levora advertisement in *U.S. Pharmacist*, September 1994.

A SHOT IN THE ARM: DEPO-PROVERA

DEPO-PROVERA (the brand name for depo-medroxyprogesterone ace-tate, or DMPA) is a synthetic progestin that suppresses ovulation, makes the cervical mucus hostile to sperm, and changes the lining of the uterus so that it will not support implantation of a fertilized egg. It is given as an injection four times a year; if you miss one shot, you must use an alternative method of contraception.

UNPLEASANT BUT EXPECTED SIDE EFFECTS

DEPO-PROVERA's side effects are similar to those of progestin-only birth control pills: breakthrough bleeding between menstrual cycles, amenorrhea, vaginal discharge, hair loss or failure to grow, hot flashes, and joint pain. At first, women using DEPO-PROVERA often experience altered menstrual patterns including irregular or unpredictable bleed-ing or spotting. By the end of the first year, however, slightly more than half of all women using DEPO-PROVERA simply stop having peri-ods; after two years, two thirds no longer menstruate.

Weight gain may be a real problem. In one study, women who used DEPO-PROVERA for two to four years gained approximately four pounds a year. These side effects disappear when use of DEPO-PRO-VERA or the pill is discontinued. The catch, of course, is that while you can just put away the pill container, once you have taken a con-traceptive injection, you are stuck with the results for at least three months.

POTENTIALLY SERIOUS ADVERSE EFFECTS

DEPO-PROVERA increases the loss of bone density, so it is considered a risk factor for osteoporosis. It also increases the risk of blood clots, stroke, and damage to the blood vessels in the eye. Clearly, if you have a personal or family history of heart disease or vascular problems, DEPO-PROVERA, like other hormonal contraceptives, is not for you.

Ditto for breast cancer. In the first four years they use DEPO-PROVERA, women younger than 35 have a risk of breast cancer slightly more than twice that of women who use other forms of contraception. The National Cancer Institute predicts an average of 27 cases of breast cancer a year for every 100,000 women aged 30 to 34. If all these women were to choose DEPO-PROVERA as their contraceptive, that rate might more than double, rising to nearly 59 cases a year for every 100,000 women in this age group.

A SECOND SHOT IN THE ARM: NORPLANT

NORPLANT is a *contraceptive system,* a group of six flexible, permeable plastic capsules containing levonorgestrel, a progestin used in several birth control pills (LEVLEN, LEVORA, NORDETTE, TRI-LEVLEN, TRIPHA-SIL). The capsules are implanted just under the skin of the upper arm and left in place for up to five years, during which time they release levonorgestrel into the body. At the end of five years, the capsules are removed and a new group may be implanted.

A RUSH OF SIDE EFFECTS

After NORPLANT was approved by the FDA in December 1990, it seemed to have a rosy future. By 1995, however, there were nearly 200 lawsuits (including 46 class-action suits) filed against Wyeth-Ayerst from women claiming that using NORPLANT had caused memory loss, muscle pain, depression, auto-immune disorders, muscle pain, depression, cancer, blood vessel problems, and heart attacks. These are similar to the side effects linked to other progestin contraceptives (see DEPO-PROVERA, above). There was also one interesting (and as yet unexplained) addition: pregnancy rates among women using NORPLANT appear to increase after three years' use among women weighing more than 150 pounds. If you are using NORPLANT, and you begin to suffer from side effects, you must return to your doctor to have the device removed.

WHAT THE DOCTORS DID

In theory, removal should be a simple process; no muss, no fuss, and quick relief. In practice, however, it has been a disaster. The physicians and technicians who put NORPLANT into 1 million American arms apparently did a bad job of it. When NORPLANT went on sale in February 1991, Wyeth-Ayerst prepared a complete set of directions on how to insert the device and how to remove it. Unfortunately, many of the people for whom the directions were intended seem not to have read them. As a result, some women discovered that the rods were implanted so deep in their arms that scar tissue had formed, making removal a nightmare. At the same time, as Barbara Seaman notes in *The Doctors' Case Against the Pill,* some U.S. judges used NORPLANT as a legal punishment. In a few well-publicized cases, women on welfare or convicted of behavior that labeled them "unfit mothers" were told to choose between using NORPLANT and either losing their benefits or going to jail.

In August 1995, stating that it found no reason to question the safety and effectiveness of a contraceptive device with a failure rate estimated at less than one percent over five years, the FDA answered complaints about NORPLANT by creating an educational campaign that includes directing doctors to disclose all potential side effects before implanting the device and offering a voluntary "patient acknowledgment form" to be signed by the patient, indicating that the doctor has told her about all NORPLANT's possible risks as well as its benefits.

CONDOMS

As they say in the song, "Everything old is new again." Especially the condom. In the age of AIDS, it is basic contraceptive equipment and first-line protection against sexually transmitted diseases.

THE BENEFITS OF CONDOMS

Condoms have lots of benefits. They are available without a prescription (the FDA is now investigating making birth control pills available over-the-counter, too). They are safe to use. And they work. When used with a spermicidal foam, they are as effective as a diaphragm plus jelly or cream. For really conscientious (and controlled) couples, who make sure the condom is on before any genital contact, and that the man withdraws immediately after ejaculation, holding the condom tight against the penis, the effectiveness of the condom/spermicide combination may approach that of the pill.

Paradoxically, condoms may also help women who *want* to become pregnant but can't. In 15 to 20 percent of all unexplained cases of infertility, the woman's body appears to manufacture antibodies to a protein on the surface of her partner's sperm. For these women, every act of unprotected intercourse triggers the immune reaction, increasing the production of antibodies. Using condoms for intercourse, often for months, until blood or cervical mucus tests show that the number of sperm antibodies has decreased and then having unprotected sex at ovulation, may increase the likelihood of pregnancy 50 to 60 percent.

In addition, latex condoms *do* protect against sexually transmitted diseases (STDs). These condoms have no pores through which viruses such as HIV may pass, which is why the government permits condom makers to advertise that their products may help prevent the spread of AIDS. Numerous studies have attested to this fact. For example, World Health Organization researchers studying whether condoms protect prostitutes in Zaire, once considered the most heavily impacted AIDS country in the world and more recently in the news as the site of the 1995 Ebola virus outbreak, found that prostitutes whose customers used condoms were AIDS-free, while those who required fewer than 25 percent of their customers to use condoms were more likely to be infected. A German study found similar results: prostitutes who used condoms were free of HIV even though they had intercourse with high-risk customers. Condoms also prevent the transmission of other STDs such as syphilis, gonorrhea, and human papilloma virus (implicated in the cause of genital warts and cervical cancer).

Warnings that condoms are not foolproof are accurate, but they are based on the facts of a condom's tearing, of its not being put on before genital contact, and of its leaking during withdrawal. According to John N. Krieger of the Department of Urology at Washington University in St. Louis, "condom breakage ratios are low (2 or less per 100 tested in the United States)." Other estimates put tears and breakage as high as 5 percent, but most experts say the fault lies with the user, not the condom.

CHOOSING A CONDOM

Standing in front of a condom display at your local drugstore, you may find it hard to believe that fewer than 20 years ago you had to sidle into the store and practically whisper your order to the druggist because most states forbade open displays of condoms.

Today, the problem isn't finding the condoms, it's finding the condom best for you. Here are some of the things to look for.

MATERIAL   The only reported side effect of condoms is an occasional allergic reaction to a lubricant or spermicide or to latex, the natural rubber product used for most American-made condoms. In the spring of 1995, the FDA approved the first allergy test for latex. The test, which measures latex antibodies in the blood, is used to identify people suspected of having an allergy to latex. It can prevent future reactions by confirming the allergy. Men or women who are sensitive to latex may switch to the polyurethane condom (AVANTI), which was approved by the FDA in 1994, or use natural skin condoms (FOUREX, NATURLAMB). Skin condoms protect against pregnancy but not against STDs. Polyurethane is assumed to protect against pregnancy and perhaps against STDs, but as of this writing, the FDA is still awaiting confirming tests.

SIZE   The standard size for an American-made condom is about 52 mm (2") wide and 188 mm (7") long. A "snug" or "slim" condom may be about 10 percent smaller; a "large" condom is about 10 percent bigger. LIFESTYLES and LIFESTYLES SPERMICIDE are slightly wider than most condoms. TROJAN RIBBED is slightly longer than most condoms. TROJAN ENZ LARGE, TROJAN MAGNUM, and TROJAN NON-LUBRICATED are also slightly longer and wider than most condoms. Skin condoms fit and feel looser than latex condoms.

SHAPE   Condoms come in two basic shapes: a straight-sided tube and a contoured tube. The contoured version, introduced nearly 30 years ago by Schmid Laboratories, fits tighter at the top and looser at the bottom to allow the tip of the penis to move around inside the condom without pulling out. PLEASURE PLUS has a slight variation on the theme, a small pocket on the underside of the condom.

THE RESERVOIR TIP   This is a safety device, a small balloonlike bump at the end of the condom that catches the ejaculate. The reservoir tip on condoms such as RAMSES EXTRA STRENGTH, TROJAN ENZ, and TOUCH (lubricated and nonlubricated) helps to protect the condom from breaking at ejaculation. Men who use condoms without reservoir tips must be careful not to insert the penis into the condom all the way to the tip. They should allow a bit of hang-over so that the end of the condom itself serves as a reservoir to provide an extra measure of protection.

THICKNESS   The primary criticism leveled at the condom is that it interferes with sensation for both partners. All major condom-producing countries except South Korea have national standards for strength and leakage. Some, including the United States, Japan, Britain, and India use a tensile strength test, in which condoms are mechanically stretched up to 7.5 times their size under pressure not less than 240 kg of force per square centimeter. Many countries also check electronically for holes. Some put condoms through a "water test," in which the sheaths must demonstrate their ability to stretch to hold a given quantity of liquid without bursting. Some inflate condoms to a critical pressure point at which defective ones burst. *Caution:* Never, absolutely never, test a condom by blowing into it or filling it with water to check for leaks before using it. In doing so, you might weaken or tear the latex.

RAMSES ULTRA THIN (plain and ribbed), SHEIK SUPER THIN, and TOUCH THIN AND ULTRA SENSITIVE are some made-in-America thinner condoms. Although much depends on how you store and handle the condom, as a general rule the thinner the condom, the more likely it is to break. The slightly thicker, nonlubricated condoms such as TROJAN and PRIME are sometimes thought to be the safest, particularly for anal intercourse. But there are no guarantees that this is true. Unlike the soft vagina, which expands to accommodate the penis, the rectum is tight and bony, and thus far more likely to tear a condom.

SURFACE TEXTURE   Textured condoms, such as EXCITA, RAMSES EXTRA RIBBED, RAMSES ULTRA THIN RIBBED, TOUCH RIBBED, and TROJAN RIBBED, have ribs or, like TROJAN ULTRA TEXTURE, "micro dots" and "spirals." PLEASURE PLUS has ribs plus a small pocket on the underside. All are designed to provide extra stimulation of vaginal tissues or the clitoris. Textured condoms are thicker than ordinary condoms.

LUBRICATION   Lubrication, in the form of silicone powder or a lotion-type liquid, offers both comfort and safety. When using a nonlubricated condom when the vagina is dry, as it may be when we have been using tampons or when we are not fully aroused, the friction of the penis against the walls of the vagina may be irritating, or it may tear at the condom or pull it off during intercourse. People who prefer unlubricated condoms—perhaps because of a sensitivity to one of the lubricants—can substitute spermicidal cream or jelly or a nonspermicidal, water-soluble lubricant such as K-Y JELLY (see Chapter 1). *Never use petroleum jelly (VASELINE) to lubricate a latex condom. It will damage the condom.*

COLOR AND SCENT   For those of us with an artistic bent, EXCITA

FIESTA, INTENSITY, and TOUCH SUNRISE COLORS are bright and cheerful. MIDNIGHT DESIRE comes in a slightly wicked stark black. RAMSES MINT SCENTED and ULTIMA MINT SCENTED are self-explanatory. Some people find the scent exciting and pleasurable, but these condoms can be irritating to sensitive individuals.

EFFECTIVENESS   When purchasing a condom for protection against STDs, read the label carefully. It can claim to protect against these only if the brand is tested in conformity with FDA guidelines. Untested brands cannot claim to protect against STDs or pregnancy. The best bet for both prevention of pregnancy and guarding against the transmission of STDs is a latex condom, whose pores (the microscopic gaps between molecules) are so small that neither sperm nor virus are likely to pass through. Skin condoms block sperm, but not the AIDS virus.

A comparison of several condoms on the market is given in the chart on pages 83–86.

COMPARING THE PRODUCTS:
A SELECTED SAMPLE OF CONDOMS

Product (Supplier)	Lubricated	Spermicide	Textured	Reservoir Tip	Other Features
LATEX CONDOMS					
EXCITA FIESTA (Schmid)	yes	no	no	yes	bright colors
EXCITA ULTRA RIBBED (Schmid)	yes	yes	yes	yes	
INTENSITY (Ansell)	no	yes	no	no	bright colors
LIFESTYLES SPERMICIDE, LUBRICATED (Ansell)	yes	yes	no	no	
LIFESTYLES VIBRA RIBBED (Ansell)	no	yes	yes	no	
MIDNIGHT DESIRE (Ansell)	yes	no	no	yes	black
PLEASURE PLUS (Reddy)	yes	no	yes	no	pouch on underside
RAMSES EXTRA RIBBED (Schmid)	yes	yes	yes	no	
RAMSES EXTRA STRENGTH (Schmid)	yes	yes	no	yes	
RAMSES MINT SCENTED (Schmid)	no	no	no	yes	scent

Product (Supplier)	Lubricated	Spermicide	Textured	Reservoir Tip	Other Features
RAMSES SENSITOL (Schmid)	yes	no	no	no	
RAMSES ULTRA THIN (Schmid)	yes	*	no	yes	
RAMSES ULTRA THIN RIBBED (Schmid)	yes	*	yes	yes	
SAXON (Safetek)	yes	no	no	no	
SHEIK SUPER THIN (Schmid)	yes	*	no	no	
SHIEK SUPER THIN RIBBED (Schmid)	yes	*	yes	no	
SHEIK SUPER THIN SPERMICIDE, LUBRICATED, RIBBED (Schmid)	yes	yes	yes	no	
TOUCH LUBRICATED (Schmid)	yes	*	no	no	
TOUCH NON-LUBRICATED (Schmid)	no	no	no	yes	
TOUCH RIBBED LUBRICATED (Schmid)	yes	no	yes	yes	

*   Comes in both spermicide and non-spermicide versions

Product (Supplier)	Lubricated	Spermicide	Textured	Reservoir Tip	Other Features
TOUCH SUNRISE COLORS (Schmid)	yes	no	no	yes	colors
TOUCH THIN AND ULTRA SENSITIVE (Schmid)	yes	no	no	no	thinner than most
TROJAN ENZ (Carter)	yes	yes	no	yes	
TROJAN MAGNUM (Carter)	yes	yes	no	no	tapered base
TROJAN NON-LUBRICATED (Carter)	no	no	no	no	
TROJAN GOLDEN RIBBED (Carter)	yes	no	yes	yes	golden color
TROJAN ULTRA TEXTURE (Carter)	yes	no	yes	yes	
ULTIMA MINT SCENTED (Big N)	no	no	no	no	mint scent
WET 'N WILD	yes	no	no	yes	
POLYURETHANE CONDOMS					
AVANTI (Schmid)	yes	no	no	no	thinner than most: these condoms transmit heat
AVANTI SUPER THIN (Schmid)	yes	no	no	no	thinner than most: these condoms transmit heat

Product (Supplier)	Lubricated	Spermicide	Textured	Reservoir Tip	Other Features
SKIN CONDOMS					
FOUREX (Schmid)	yes	no	no	no	do not protect against many STDs
FOUREX WITH SPERMICIDE (Schmid)	yes	yes	no	no	do not protect against many STDs
NATURLAMB (Carter)	yes	no	no	no	do not protect against many STDs

Sources: Products on sale in New York City, summer 1995. Consumer information from Schmid and Ansell.

FEMALE CONDOMS

At this writing, there is only one female condom. REALITY is a dispos-able, loose-fitting polyurethane tube, closed at one end, with a flexible ring, something like the rim of a diaphragm, at each end. The ring at the closed end is inserted into the vagina; the other hangs outside so that the open end of the tube covers the outer lips of the vagina. If you have used a diaphragm, you will find it a cinch to insert REALITY, even though the closed end of the condom is slightly lighter and more flexible and bouncy than a diaphragm.

If you haven't used a diaphragm, your best bet is to practice in-serting a REALITY condom a few times by yourself without the pres-sure of immanent love-making. You can use the same REALITY condom more than once when you are practicing, but you must not use the condom more than once when you have sex. You don't need a spermi-cide when using REALITY, although the first time you try the device it's probably a good idea to use one as back up. Do not use a female condom in conjunction with a male condom because the friction be-tween them may dislodge REALITY. If you have trouble inserting the female condom or if your partner complains of dryness, you can add either the nonspermicidal lubricant that comes in the package or any lubricant you prefer.*

In use, REALITY feels different from a male condom. It covers the wall of the vagina, not the penis itself which moves freely inside the female condom. (Some male condoms attempt to create this sensation by making the condom looser through the section that covers the shaft of the penis.) REALITY's second virtue is that polyurethane, un-like latex, transmits heat, so the penis feels the temperature change as the vaginal tissues warm up during sexual arousal. As a result, in an 1995 article for *Men's Fitness* rating the "best feeling" condoms, televi-sion writer and stand-up comic Lee Frank scored REALITY in a first-place tie with the male condom PLEASURE PLUS.

REALITY may be inserted up to eight hours before having sex but must be removed right after sex, *before you stand up,* to avoid any leak-age of seminal fluid.

---

* Petroleum jelly, which damages latex condoms, will not affect this polyure-thane sheath, but it is not water soluble, which means it is a real job to remove.

PREVENTING PREGNANCY

The basic study used to predict failure (pregnancy) rates for the female condom was a six-month trial in 1990 in the United States and Latin America. The study was conducted jointly by the Family Health International in Research Triangle Park, North Carolina, and the Contraceptive Research and Development Program. They recruited 377 women aged 18 to 40 who were engaged in mutually monogamous heterosexual relationships and were willing to use the female condom as their only form of birth control for six months.

At the end of the study, the overall failure rate (number of pregnancies) in typical use was 15 percent; in the United States, 12.4 percent. To establish an annual failure rate, the FDA simply doubled the six-month rate to 25 percent, suggesting that one of every four women using REALITY for one year will become pregnant. This information appears on the REALITY package.

However, many contraceptive researchers question the accuracy of this statistic. For one thing, birth control research generally shows that as people become more familiar with a method, the failure rate tends to drop. For another, the *overall* failure rate may not reflect the true incidence of failure among women who use the female condom correctly and every time they have sex. Indeed, when they reexamined the trial numbers, eliminating women who used the female condom only once in a while, a team of scientists led by James Trussell, professor of economics and public affairs and associate dean at the Woodrow Wilson School of Public Affairs and director of the Office of Popular Research at Princeton University, found that the failure rates dropped dramatically, to 2.6 per 100 U.S. women. Their conclusion? The "true" annual failure rate for the female condom in "typical use" may actually be 19 to 25 percent, higher than in the study, but the failure rate in "perfect use" (among women who use the device precisely as directed, every time they have sex) may be around 5 percent, only slightly higher than the 3 percent "perfect use" failure rate for male condoms.

PROTECTING AGAINST DISEASE

For ethical reasons, it was impossible to test whether the polyurethane REALITY sheath protects against HIV transmission during sex. No contraceptive is 100 percent effective against sexually transmitted diseases, but Trussell has written that using the female condom would reduce the odds of acquiring the AIDS virus to one chance in 167 for a woman who has sex with an infected male partner twice a week for one year. The FDA permits the REALITY package to carry these words: "Intended to provide protection against pregnancy and sexually transmitted disease, including AIDS (HIV infection)."

DIAPHRAGMS

Using a mechanical barrier inside the vagina to keep sperm from reaching the uterus is not a new idea. The earliest diaphragms were probably firm fruit shells, such as half a hollowed-out lemon or pomegranate. As you might imagine, none of these fit as snugly or comfortably as a modern diaphragm, so they were nowhere near as protective, although they were probably better than nothing at all because the naturally acid fruit juices may have had at least a minimal spermicidal effect.

Luckily, modern diaphragms fit better, feel better, and work much more reliably to prevent pregnancy. We can sit around all night swapping stories about the diaphragm's effectiveness, but the statistics are straightforward: if 100 women use the diaphragm with spermicide for one year, as few as 3 or as many as 18 may become pregnant. However, there are countless women who have used a diaphragm for 20 years or more to successfully prevent or space pregnancies. Its effectiveness clearly depends in large measure on our doctors' willingness to take the time to fit the diaphragm correctly and teach us how it works, and our own willingness to use it properly.

If a diaphragm is too large, it may hurt when a partner's penis pushes it against the bladder during intercourse. If it is too large or too small, it may not fit snugly behind the pubic bone and may slip out of place. To ensure that your diaphragm is the correct size, it makes sense to visit your doctor for a new fitting once a year, or when you gain or lose more than ten pounds, have a baby, or have a miscarriage or an abortion.

HOW TO USE A DIAPHRAGM

Before inserting your diaphragm, hold it up to the light and check for holes. Then, urinate to empty your bladder so that it is less likely to be uncomfortable when you have intercourse. Using a diaphragm may increase the risk of a urinary tract infection because it may press on the bladder, preventing you from emptying it completely and allowing a pool of urine to remain in the bladder and offer a place for bacteria to multiply. Bacteria may also enter the urinary tract when you insert the diaphragm or when you remove it, or when it is left in place longer than the six hours recommended.

To reduce the risk, wash your hands before inserting or removing the diaphragm. Be sure to use a sufficient amount of spermicidal cream or jelly—a teaspoonful inside the cup, a slick coating around the rim and on the outside of the cup—but not so much that the diaphragm will slip out of your fingers when you try to insert it. Once the diaphragm is in place, check to see that it is covering the cervix, which you may feel as a bump right behind the middle of the cup. Without reaching in to check this, you cannot be certain that the diaphragm is protecting the cervix from sperm.

For maximum protection, you must use the diaphragm *every single time you have intercourse,* including days when you are sure you are not fertile. This simple rule cannot be overemphasized.

After intercourse, leave the diaphragm in place for 6 hours. If you wish to have intercourse again during that time, use an applicator to insert a second application of spermicide such as foam or cream. Insert the spermicide *without removing the diaphragm*. Or have your partner use a condom.

It is best to remove the diaphragm as soon as possible once 6 hours have passed, although you may leave it in longer if you have had intercourse again during the 6 hours. However, you should *never* leave the diaphragm in place for longer than 24 hours. The surface of the diaphragm, nestled deep in the vaginal canal, provides a hospitable environment for certain pathogens, bacteria that cause disease. There have been some reports that women who wear diaphragms for long periods of time may be at higher risk of toxic shock syndrome, the potentially fatal infection originally linked to super-absorbent menstrual tampons (see page 46–49).

When you remove the diaphragm, wash it, dry it thoroughly, and store it in its case.

Clearly, to use a diaphragm safely and successfully, it helps to be the kind of woman one group of researchers has described as "intelligent, motivated, conscientious, and perhaps, somewhat obsessive."*

---

* Charles E. Flowers Jr., Lee R. Beck, and Walter H. Wilborn, "The contraceptive aspects of the anatomy, morphology, and physiology of the vagina," *Vaginal Contraception* (New York: Harper and Row, 1979), 20.

The reward for your persistence will be an effective contraceptive without the side effects associated with chemicals or IUDs.

BRANDS AND TYPES OF DIAPHRAGMS

There are three basic types of diaphragms, all of which are natural rubber (ORTHO) or rubber latex (KORO-FLEX, KOROMEX), each named for the type of wire inside the rim.

COIL SPRING DIAPHRAGMS   These diaphragms (KOROMEX COIL SPRING, ORTHO COIL SPRING) have a thin spiral metal wire inside the rim. This spring bends easily in every direction, but it is very bouncy—coil spring diaphragms have been know to leap from the hands of women trying to insert them and end up halfway across the room. However, this very bounciness has distinct advantages for women who have

- very firm vaginal muscles; if the muscles are not firm, they may fold in around the rim of the diaphragm, making it difficult to remove

- an upright uterus that does not tilt either forward or back

- a deep arc in the vagina right behind the pubic bone, the space your doctor feels during a pelvic examination when he or she reaches upward toward the surface of the abdomen

FLAT SPRING DIAPHRAGMS   These (ORTHO-WHITE FLAT SPRING) have a flat metal spring, something like a watch spring. Like the coil spring diaphragm, these may also be too flexible for women with weak vaginal muscles, but they work well for women with

- firm vaginal muscles

- a uterus tilted slightly forward ("anteflex")

- a shallow arc behind the pubic bone

- a long curved cervix, pointing slightly backward

ARCING SPRING DIAPHRAGM   These (KORO-FLEX ARCING SPRING, ORTHO ALL FLEX), have a very firm rim that allows you to fold the diaphragm neatly in half for insertion. These diaphragms are very easy to insert and work well for women who have

- flabby vaginal muscles; the firm rim pushes back the vaginal walls so that the diaphragm is easy to remove even if you have poor muscle tone; if your vaginal muscles are firm the arcing spring diaphragm will be uncomfortable because it does not yield when the vaginal walls contract during orgasm

- cystocele (a protrusion of the bladder wall into the vagina, usually resulting from a tear in the vaginal muscle during childbirth) or rectocele (a protrusion of the rectal wall into the vagina)

- a retroverted (backward tilting) uterus

WHY DO DIAPHRAGMS FAIL?

As one major contraceptive textbook says, "The greatest detriment to successful diaphragm use is combining it with rhythm."* That is, not using it every time you have intercourse.

But it is also true that diaphragms fail even when users do everything right. When a woman is sexually aroused, her vagina balloons slightly, and a diaphragm that fits perfectly when she is not aroused may slip for a minute. If that happens just as her partner ejaculates— that is, if they have simultaneous orgasms—some sperm may sprint around the diaphragm and enter the cervix. In *Women and the Crisis in Sex Hormones,* medical writer Barbara Seaman suggests that women for whom the diaphragm is consistently an effective birth control method may succeed simply because their orgasm occurs before their partners ejaculate so that by the time the sperm are released into the vagina, the diaphragm is safely back in place, snug around the cervix.

Finally, if you choose to use a diaphragm, it is important to remember that while it covers the cervix, it does not offer protection against sexually transmitted disease, including AIDS, which spread through contact with the mucous membrane lining of the vagina.

CERVICAL CAPS

A cervical cap is a rubber latex device about the size of a thimble. It comes in four standard sizes designed to fit snugly over the cervix

---

* Charles E. Flowers Jr., Lee R. Beck, and Walter H. Wilborn, "The contraceptive aspects of the anatomy, morphology, and physiology of the vagina," *Vaginal Contraception* (New York: Harper and Row, 1979), 20.

where it is held in place by suction. Once regarded as a contraceptive that could be left in place throughout the month, the cervical cap is now meant to be inserted right before intercourse and removed about eight hours later. It can safely remain in place for two days. It takes practice to be able to use a cervical cap; like the diaphragm, it provides no protection against sexually transmitted disease.

CONTRACEPTIVE SPONGES

The TODAY contraceptive sponge, a barrier contraceptive with spermicide, was introduced in 1983 and sold without a prescription for the next 11 years. Early in 1994, however, an FDA inspection of the Whitehall-Robins plant in New Jersey where the sponge was made found a type of diarrhea bacteria in the plant's water system. No contamination of the sponges was ever found, but the FDA tightened the standards for measuring water purity to a level the company believed unreasonable. Unable to come to an agreement with the FDA, Whitehall ceased production of the TODAY sponge in 1995.

IUDS

The very first IUDs were almost certainly the pebbles that nomadic Arabs inserted into the uteruses of female camels to keep them from becoming pregnant during long treks across the desert. The pebbles worked because they made it uncomfortable for the animals to mate.

In 1891, an English gynecology textbook reported the large number of "pessaries" in use for human beings, describing elastic catheters with flexible wire stylets used as early as 1803 and later models including those with an ivory stem. There was some question, however, about whether these were used for contraception or, as the writer put it, to counteract "all flexions of the uterus," that is, to keep the uterus straight and upright in the abdomen. The first contraceptive intrauterine device was the Grafenberg rings made of silver or silkworm gut and placed in the uterus after dilating the cervix.

Modern IUDs, which are inserted in a similar fashion, are recommended only for women who have delivered at least one child, have no history of pelvic inflammatory disease, no uterine or cervical cancer, no undiagnosed vaginal bleeding, no history of ectopic pregnancy, no untreated vaginal infection, and—because they do not prevent sexually transmitted disease—have a stable, monogamous sexual relationship.

TYPES OF IUDS

There are two types of IUDs, the LIPPES LOOP and the PARAGARD T380A.

The LIPPES LOOP is a plain polyethylene device shaped like a double S. It comes in four sizes to accommodate the normal variations in the size of the human uterus: Loop A (22.2 mm) is for women who need a smaller IUD. Loop B (27.5 mm) has smaller curves to the S and is for women who have either suffered miscarriage or have a small uterus. Loop C (30 mm) has even smaller curves to the S and is for women who seemed able to accommodate a Loop D but had it removed because of pain or bleeding. Loop D (33 mm) is for women who have had one or more children.

All four sizes have a fine, double polyethylene thread attached to the lower end. This thread hangs out through the cervix, allowing you to check that the IUD is still in place (women sometimes expel them spontaneously) and, if necessary, facilitates removal.

No one is certain exactly how the polyethylene IUD prevents pregnancy, but one theory is that it stimulates a "foreign body" reaction that makes the walls of the uterus inhospitable to a fertilized egg.

The PARAGARD T380A is the third generation of copper IUDs. It is shaped (as its name implies) like a T, with each arm 32 mm long. Like the LIPPES LOOP, the PARAGARD is made of polyethylene with a microfilament polyethylene thread tied to the bottom. What makes it different is that its arms are wrapped in copper, 176 mg on the upright stem, a copper collar at the center of the cross bar, and 665 mg. on each arm. In addition, it contains barium sulfate, which makes it "radiopaque" so that it is visible on X-ray.

It is also unclear exactly how copper prevents conception. Studies suggest that the copper may reduce the number of viable sperm in the vaginal tract, interfere with the sperm's ability to penetrate the egg, or interfere with a fertilized egg's ability to implant in the uterine wall.

RISKS OF IUDS

IUDs have been known to perforate (tear) the cervix or the uterus during insertion and have been linked to cramping, weakness, and dizziness just after they are put in place. There may also be bleeding and cramping for a few days after your doctor inserts an IUD. While you are using an IUD, your periods may be heavier than normal, so that you lose more blood and need to take iron supplements.

While using an IUD, the risk of pelvic inflammatory disease (PID) is three to five times higher than it would be with another form of contraception, perhaps because the thread hanging down through the cervix provides a ladder on which bacteria can ascend into the uterus. The DALKON SHIELD, implicated in the majority of injuries and illnesses associated with earlier versions of the IUD, differed from other intrauterine devices in that it had a many-threaded tail that might have increased the possibility of infection. Occasionally, an IUD may become embedded in the uterine wall. If this happens, the IUD must be removed surgically.

Copper IUDs present some unique problems. For one thing, using one may cause a skin rash if you are allergic to the metal. If you have Wilson's disease, a disorder that leads to higher-than-normal concentrations of copper in the body, using a copper IUD may exacerbate your symptoms. Short-wave or microwave medical diathermy may make the copper hot enough to cause internal burns. But studies show that women using a copper IUD suffer no ill effects from magnetic resonance imaging (MRI).

ARE IUDS EFFECTIVE?

Some women using IUDs conceive because their bodies expel the devices without warning. Others become pregnant with their IUDs firmly in place. Such conceptions are associated with a higher incidence of ectopic pregnancy, in which the fertilized egg implants in the Fallopian tube or some other site outside the uterus. If the egg implants in the tube, the growing fetus must be removed surgically because it would eventually rupture the tube. Even a uterine pregnancy with an IUD in place is dangerous and may result in serious complications including septic (infected) abortion, a miscarriage accompanied by an infection in the blood that may be fatal to both mother and child.

When a woman has an IUD removed, she is generally (but not always) able to become pregnant. In one study of 293 women, 78.4 percent seeking to become pregnant succeeded in the first year after removal.

For a table on the rate of effectiveness of IUDs see page 96.

COMPARING THE PRODUCTS:
HOW EFFECTIVE ARE IUDS?

If 100 women use this device for one year	...this many will decide to continue to use the device	...this many are likely to experience pregnancy	...and this many are likely to experience expulsion of their IUD
PARAGARD T380A (GynaPharma)	79.6	0.5–0.6*	5.3–5.7
LIPPES LOOP A (Ortho)	75.2	5.3[†]	23.9
LIPPES LOOP B (Ortho)	74.6	3.4	18.9
LIPPES LOOP C (Ortho)	76.5	3.0	19.1
LIPPES LOOP D (Ortho)	77.4	2.7	12.7

* The results for PARAGARD are reported in terms of two numbers. The first number is for women who have had children; the second number is for all women using the device.

† The results for the LIPPES LOOPS are for all women using the product.

Source: Physicians' Desk Reference, 46th ed. (Montvale, NJ: Medical Economics Data, 1992).

SPERMICIDES

Among upper-class women of the twelfth dynasty in ancient Egypt, around 1850 B.C., elephant and crocodile dung, honey and soda, and various gum substances were used to block the vagina during intercourse. The Ebers papyrus (the first written medical record) dated around 1500 B.C. contains a prescription for lint tampons moistened with fermented acacia juice. Aristotle recommended using oil to cover the cervix and coat the lining of the vagina.

Did they work? Maybe. Sticky substances such as honey and dung would clump the sperm and slow them down, while the alkaline dung and the acidic acacia juice would change the environment of the vagina so as to make it less hospitable to the sperm. Oil would indeed cover the cervix and again slow down the sperm.

But for serious contraception, modern products have them beat hands down. Contraceptive jellies, creams, foam, foaming tablets, and vaginal suppositories work by inactivating sperm so that they cannot travel up through the cervix into the uterus and on to a rendezvous with the egg. These OTC products are easy to use and they are a good backup to other contraceptives, particularly condoms and when you have missed a birth control pill. To be effective, they must form a protective barrier across the cervix. Creams and foams do this more effectively than jellies, tablets, or suppositories.

Currently, all chemical barrier contraceptives contain either nonoxynol-9 or octoxynol-9, surfactants that are rarely irritating, although some men, particularly those with light skin, hair, and eyes, may be sensitive to it. An allergic reaction might include irritation, burning, or itching in the genital area.

Nonoxynol-9 spermicides may offer some protection against sexually transmitted disease including gonorrhea, chlamydia, several forms of vaginitis, and genital herpes. There is no conclusive evidence to show that they protect against AIDS. On the other hand, they may make a woman more susceptible to urinary infections because the spermicide kills off "good" bacteria in the vagina, allowing potentially harmful *E. coli* to flourish. Women who get frequent urinary infections should discuss their contraceptives with their doctors.

As with condoms and diaphragms, the effectiveness of contraceptive jellies, creams, inserts, and suppositories depends on how single-minded you are about using them, although vaginal tablets do not offer the same protection as the others. Today, most manufacturers recommend using a spermicide with a condom or diaphragm for maximum effectiveness. And one thing more: like all drug and cosmetics products, spermicides have an expiration date. Observe it—and keep the products at room temperature, neither too hot nor too cool. A bedside table is perfect.

GELS, JELLIES, AND CREAMS

These are generally meant to be used with a diaphragm or condom. If the product can be used alone, use two doses for maximum protection against pregnancy. Creams, gels, and jellies provide extra lubrication during intercourse; both may leak from the vagina; both are water soluble and wash off easily. Personal preference will dictate whether you like the texture of one more than the other; the creams feel like light lotions. Gels and jellies have a similar slick texture, but jellies are lighter. The lighter creams leak more easily. Be sure to keep these products out of the reach of children; large amounts may be toxic if swallowed by a small child. Small amounts are safe for an adult engaging in oral sex.

One new product with an interesting twist is ADVANTAGE 24 (Johnson & Johnson), a bioadhesive gel designed to adhere to the walls of the vagina. It does not leak, can be inserted up to 24 hours in advance, and comes in individually wrapped prefilled applicators

FOAMS

Contraceptive foams are spermicidal creams packed in aerosol containers which fluff up the products as they are released from the cans into the applicators. Early on, foam had a reputation as a risky contraceptive. The reason? Early tests of foams were almost uniformly discouraging, with as many as 30 of every 100 women using foam for one year becoming pregnant. However, it turned out that many women did not know how to use the foam or were not motivated to use it every time they had sex.

Later tests among women who were properly instructed and motivated show that foam approaches 100 percent effectiveness in preventing pregnancy. Doubling the dose improves protection, and using it with a condom produces a contraceptive method every bit as good as a diaphragm used with spermicide. In one study, the condom/foam combination had no failure rate at all. Foam is not meant to be inserted into a diaphragm, as it may not adhere to the rim and outside of the latex. But you can insert it after you put in the diaphragm, or use it as a backup if you engage in intercourse within six hours after putting the diaphragm in place. (One application of cream or jelly is good for only one episode of intercourse.) Foam disperses quickly and may also offer some minimal protection against sexually transmitted diseases.

TABLETS AND SUPPOSITORIES

These are the least effective contraceptive products. All require at least 15 minutes or longer to dissolve or liquefy into a protective film. One 1979 study of a vaginal tablet showed it still intact even after 15 minutes in 6 of the 20 women who were testing it. In addition, one study in the late 1970s showed that in the United States, the failure rate (number of pregnancies) for vaginal tablets and suppositories might be as high as 40 percent (that is, 40 of every 100 women who used them for one year got pregnant).

If you use one of these products and wish to douche, wait six hours after intercourse.

For a table comparing a selection of topical vaginal spermicides see pages 100–102.

COMPARING THE PRODUCTS:
TOPICAL VAGINAL SPERMICIDES

Product (Supplier)	Type	Features*
ADVANTAGE 24 (Lake)	gel	"Bioadhesive": it clings to vaginal walls and may be applied up to 24 hours before intercourse. May be used alone or with a condom. Packed in prefilled applicators.
CONCEPTROL (Ortho/Advanced Care Products)	gel	Apply at least 10 minutes before having intercourse to allow gel to disperse evenly throughout the vagina. May be used alone or with a condom. Packed in prefilled applicators. Questions? Call 1-800-652-6532
CONCEPTROL (Ortho/Advanced Care Products)	inserts	Tablet may require 15 minutes after insertion to dissolve in a normally moist vagina. If vaginal tissues are dry, it may take longer. Protection lasts 1 hour. If you wish to have intercourse a second time, use a second insert. Repeat as frequently as required. May be used alone or with a condom or as a second application of spermicide with a diaphragm.[†] Questions? Call 1-800-652-6532
DELFEN (Ortho/Advanced Care Products)	foam	May be inserted immediately before intercourse. May be used alone or with condom or as a second application of spermicide with a diaphragm.[†] Unscented. Questions? Call 1-800-652-6532

Product (Supplier)	Type	Features*
ENCARE (Thompson Medical)	supposi-tory	Suppository requires at least 10 minutes to dissolve in vagina. Protection lasts 1 hour. If you wish to have intercourse a second time, use a second suppository. Repeat as frequently as required. May be used alone or with a condom or as a second application of spermicide with a diaphragm.[†] Unscented. Package insert printed in English and Spanish.
GYNOL II (Ortho/Advanced Care Products)	jelly	For use with a diaphragm. Protection lasts 6 hours. If you have intercourse a second time within 6 hours, insert a second application.[†] May be used with a condom. Unscented. Questions? Call: 1-800-652-6532
GYNOL II EXTRA STRENGTH (Ortho/Advanced Care Products)	jelly	Higher concentration of spermicide than GYNOL II.
KOROMEX (Gyna Pharma/Schmid)	cream*	For use with a diaphragm or condom.
KOROMEX (Gyna Phrama/Schmid)	gel	For use with a diaphragm or condom. Unscented.
KOROMEX (Gyna Pharma/Schmid)	jelly	May be used alone or with a diaphragm or condom.
KOROMEX (Gyna Pharma/Schmid)	foam	May be inserted immediately before intercourse. May be used alone or with a condom or as a second application of spermicide with a diaphragm.[†]

Product (Supplier)	Type	Features*
K-Y PLUS (Johnson & Johnson)	jelly	For use with a condom. Protection lasts 1 hour after insertion. Unscented. Provides lubrication plus spermicide. This product may be especially useful for women approaching menopause when vaginal tissues begin to thin and dry. DO NOT CONFUSE THIS PRODUCT WITH PLAIN K-Y JELLY, WHICH CONTAINS NO SPERMICIDE AND IS NOT A CONTRACEPTIVE PRODUCT. Questions? Call 1-800-526-3967
ORTHO GYNOL (Ortho/Advanced Care Products)	jelly	see GYNOL II
SEMICID (Whitehall)	supposi-tory	Requires at least 10 minutes to dissolve in vagina. Protection lasts 1 hour. If you wish to have intercourse a second time, use a second suppository. Repeat as frequently as required. May be used alone or with a condom or as a second application of spermicide with a diaphragm.[†] Unscented. Questions? Call 1-800-883-3279

* The spermicide in all products in this list except KOROMEX cream is nonoxynol-9. The spermicide in KOROMEX cream is octoxynol-9. Both are rated safe and effective for contraception.

† When using as a second application, insert *without* removing diapragm.

Sources: Products on sale in New York City, summer 1995. *Physicians' Desk Reference for Nonprescription Drugs*, 16th ed. (Montvale, NJ: Medical Economics Data, 1995). Roberta S. Carrier, "Contraceptive methods and products," *Handbook of Nonprescription Drugs*, 9th ed. (Washington, DC: American Pharmaceutical Association, 1990).

NATURAL FAMILY PLANNING

Women who wish to avoid pregnancy but do not want to use chemical or mechanical contraceptives may turn to natural family planning, a form of birth control based on avoiding intercourse during ovulation, the one time during the menstrual cycle when contraception can occur.

THE CALENDAR METHOD

This is the simplest but least reliable method of natural family planning. It requires a woman to chart her menstrual cycles on a year-long calendar, which is used to help identify a menstrual pattern. A woman with absolutely regular 28-day cycles could predict her time of ovulation. Knowing that sperm can live for several days inside the female reproductive tract, that the egg released at ovulation can live up to 24 hours after it leaves the ovary, and that, finally, a woman might—though rarely—release a second egg, this woman would avoid pregnancy by avoiding intercourse for 5 days prior to ovulation and 3 days after. The catch is that any deviation from the 28-day cycle complicates the process. If cycles are truly irregular—28 days one month, 32 the next—it is virtually impossible for a woman to predict when her ovulation will occur.

THE TEMPERATURE METHOD

This type of family planning is based on the fact that when we ovulate, our bodies produce a sudden burst of progesterone that sends our body temperature up a few tenths of a degree. Measuring your temperature on a special "ovulation thermometer" marked to show these small differences in tenths of a degree from 96°F to 100°F allows you to see the change. In the middle of the menstrual cycle, when your temperature rises and remains high for a few days, it is reasonable to assume that ovulation has occurred. The temperature method requires abstaining from intercourse until three days after ovulation. However, you should be aware that an illness, no matter how minor, or even a few days of tension at home or at the office can play havoc with temperature readings and, occasionally, with ovulation itself.

THE MUCUS METHOD

This third form of natural family planning requires you to observe changes in vaginal secretions during the menstrual cycle. After menstrual bleeding stops, the vaginal mucus is scant and sticky. Right before ovulation, as estrogen secretion increases, there is an increased production of vaginal mucus that feels slippery, stretchy, and wet, rather like raw egg white. This mucus is full of sugars and trace elements needed for sperm survival and to increase the sperm's ability to swim up to the egg. Shortly after ovulation the secretions decrease or become sticky once again.

To use the mucus method effectively, you have to be sufficiently at ease with your body that you can watch, perhaps touch, and evaluate the mucus. If you choose to use this method of natural family planning, remember that several things can affect the consistency of the vaginal secretions, including: vaginal infections, sexual arousal, sperm deposited in the vagina during intercourse, and medications such as antihistamines and decongestants, which dry mucous membranes in the vagina as well as the respiratory tract.

The advantages of the mucus method are that it is readily available, cheap, and reliable if you are willing to comply with all the requirements. In one 1982 study of 19,843 fertile women in Calcutta, the failure rate of the mucus method of natural family planning was comparable to that of the pill: 0.2 pregnancies per 100 women using the method for one year. A similar result was found in a 1984 study of German women, with a pregnancy rate of 0.8 per 100 women using the method for one year.

See page 105 for a comparison of the effectiveness of the most common natural family planning methods.

COMPARING THE EFFECTIVENESS
OF NATURAL FAMILY PLANNING METHODS

If 100 women use this method for one year	...this many will become pregnant
The calendar method	14–47
The temperature method	1–20
The mucus method	1–20
The temperature method plus the mucus method with intercourse only after ovulation	fewer than 1–7
No method at all	60–80

Source: "Contraception: Comparing the options," HEW Publication No. (FDA) 73-3069.

CHOOSING A CONTRACEPTIVE

The method of contraception you use must fit your personal requirements. First, if you are postponing pregnancy but would not really mind having a child if your birth control fails, you have more leeway than if medical considerations make it absolutely imperative that you not become pregnant. Second, if you and your partner are monogamous, the contraceptive you choose does not necessarily have to protect you from sexually transmitted diseases. The charts on the next two pages rank birth control methods according to their relative ability to prevent pregnancy and protect against STDs. The chart on page 108 gives statistics on the mortality rates related to different birth-control methods.

COMPARING THE EFFECTIVENESS
OF CONTRACEPTIVE METHODS

If 100 women use this method for one year	. . . the lowest expected number of pregnancies is*	. . . the typical reported number of pregnancies is
Injection (Depo-Provera)	less than 1	less than 1
Implant (Norplant)	less than 1	less than 1
Sterilization (male or female)	less than 1	less than 1
Oral contraceptive	less than 1	3
IUD (copper)	less than 1	3[†]
Condom	2	12
Diaphragm w/ spermicide**	3	18
Withdrawal	4	18
Natural birth control (all methods of periodic abstinence)	1–10	20
Spermicide alone**	3	21
Female condom	††	††
No contraceptive method	85–89	85–89

* These rates are for the first continuous year of use; ranges reflect differing assessments from different sources.

† For all types of IUDs

** Foams, creams, jellies, or suppositories, used exactly as directed

†† In its first 6 months of use, the failure rate for the female condom was 12.5 pregnancies for every 100 women. As of this writing, the FDA has interpreted this to mean that the annual failure rate will be 25 pregnancies (twice 12.5). A number of experts dispute this figure, maintaining that effectiveness increases with familiarity. According to the company's research, the actual annual failure rate with REALITY is 2.5 pregnancies for every 100 women; other studies put it slightly higher, around five percent (see pages 87–88).

DOES YOUR CONTRACEPTIVE PROTECT AGAINST SEXUALLY TRANSMITTED DISEASE?

Method	Protection
Male latex condom	Very good
Female condom	Very good
Diaphragm	Fair
Cervical cap	Fair
Spermicide	Fair
IUD	None
Oral contraceptive	None
Injection (Depo-Provera)	None
Implant (Norplant)	None

Sources (for table on page 106 and above): Package insert for DEPO-PROVERA and REALITY on sale, summer 1995. Roberta S. Carrier, *Handbook of Nonprescription Drugs*, 9th ed. (Washington, DC: American Pharmaceutical Association, 1990). *Physicians' Desk Reference*, 48th ed. (Montvale, NJ: Medical Economics Data, 1994). "Condoms, contraceptives and STDs. Does your birth control method protect you from sexually transmitted disease?" (Triangle Research Park, NC: American Social Health Association, 1994). John N. Krieger, "New sexually transmitted disease treatment guidelines," *Journal of Urology*, July 1995.

IS YOUR CONTRACEPTIVE SAFE?

NUMBER OF WOMEN'S DEATHS EACH YEAR RELATED TO CHILDBIRTH OR TO A SPECIFIC METHOD OF BIRTH CONTROL

Method	Deaths per 100,000 fertile women by age group					
	15–19	20–24	25–29	30–34	35–39	40–44
Method-related deaths						
Oral contraceptive (nonsmokers)	0.3	0.5	0.9	1.9	13.8	31.6
Oral contraceptive (smokers)	2.2	3.4	6.6	13.5	51.1	117.2
IUD	0.8	0.8	1.0	1.0	1.4	1.4
Childbirth-related deaths						
Condom	1.1	1.6	0.7	0.2	0.3	0.4
Diaphragm w/ spermicide	1.9	1.2	1.2	1.3	2.2	2.8
Natural birth control (all methods of periodic abstinence)	2.5	1.6	1.6	1.7	2.9	3.6
No contraceptive method	7.0	7.4	9.1	14.8	25.7	28.2

Source: Physicians' Desk Reference, 48th ed. (Montvale, NJ: Medical Economics Data, 1994).

CONTRACEPTION AFTER THE FACT

FOLK REMEDIES

As long as there have been old wives, there have been old wives' tales about plants and herbs that "bring on your period," a euphemism for terminating an unwanted pregnancy. It is important to realize that any product we use as an abortifacient deserves the respect accorded all medications. Simply because they are "natural" does not mean that plants and their chemicals are harmless. Plants containing chemicals effective enough to cause uterine contractions that expel a fetus are strong enough to cause other problems such as liver or kidney failure. The bottom line: no plant or herbal remedy should be used to end a pregnancy.

SOME THINGS THAT OFFER MINIMAL PROTECTION

Spermicidal jellies, creams, and foam inserted *immediately* after inter-course may lend some protection in an emergency—for example, when a condom breaks or spills. But none is as effective after intercourse as it is before; if they're handy enough to use after the damage is done, so to speak, they're handy enough to use properly before the event.

THE MORNING-AFTER PILL

As long ago as 1980, a study from the National Institutes of Health showed that women given ethinyl estradiol (the estrogen in birth con-trol pills) or conjugated estrogens (the estrogen used for menopausal hormone replacement therapy) within 72 hours of unprotected inter-course had a reduced incidence of pregnancy of 85 percent.

Today, the American College of Obstetricians and Gynecologists (ACOG) explains that estrogens protect by delivering hormones that prevent the uterine lining from preparing for implantation. The "morning-after pill," says ACOG, is the birth control pill that may be effective 60 to 90 percent of the time.

Most gynecologists, but not most women, know that the pill can also be used as a morning-after pill, says a 1995 study from Kaiser Family Foundation in Menlo Park, California. The pill often causes nausea and vomiting, but, says Dr. James Trussell of Princeton University, author of *Emergency Contraception: The Nation's Best Kept Secret*, it also may prevent as many as 75 percent of pregnancies that would otherwise occur.

Unlike RU-486, the French drug that induces abortion in the early weeks of pregnancy and is currently being tested as an emergency contraceptive in the United States, the hormones in birth control pills prevent the fertilized egg from implanting in the lining of the uterus. According to ACOG, taking two 0.05 mg estrogen/0.5 mg progestin combination pills within 72 hours of unprotected sex and repeating the dose 12 hours later appears to significantly reduce the risk of pregnancy. In 1996, the FDA approved this use and granted permission for manufacturers to include the pertinent information in product inserts.*

A copper IUD inserted seven to ten days after unprotected intercourse may also provide morning-after protection. Although most doctors say they would provide such help, they rarely do. One reason, the Kaiser study said, is that women may not know enough to ask for it. Six of ten American women have heard of emergency contraception, but only 20 percent know that it is effective as long as 72 hours (three days) after intercourse.

INFERTILITY

For most of us, birth control means finding a way to prevent pregnancy. For people who are infertile, controlling reproduction often means searching desperately for a way to become pregnant.

Infertility is not a term to be applied lightly. It means that a female has failed to conceive after a full year of intercourse without contraception with a partner whose sperm are capable of fertilizing an egg.

There are many reasons why women may be infertile. Those who have used oral contraceptives sometimes have difficulty conceiving when they stop. Scarring from a sexually transmitted disease may block the fallopian tubes, preventing an egg from descending to meet the sperm. Hormonal problems may interfere with ovulation or prevent a fertilized egg from implanting in the uterus.

If a woman's doctor determines that her infertility is due to a failure to ovulate, he or she may prescribe one of the drugs on the following pages.

---

* Low-dose pills (0.035 mg estrogen) may also be effective, but this regimen has not yet been evaluated.

DRUGS USED TO TREAT FEMALE INFERTILITY CAUSED BY FAILURE TO OVULATE

Brand Name (Supplier)	Generic Name	Product Information
CLOMID (Marion Merrell Dow)	Clomiphene citrate (tablet)	**How it works:** Clomiphene citrate stimulates production of LH and FSH, pituitary hormones that signal the ovary to produce and release an egg (ovulation). It is used to treat infertility caused by a lack of these hormones. **How well it succeeds:** Of 5,154 patients treated with clomiphene citrate, 75 percent ovulated; 35–46 percent become pregnant; 14 percent suffered a miscarriage. **Multiple births/birth defects:** 10 percent of the women who become pregnant while using this drug have multiple fetuses; less than 1 percent have 3 or more fetuses. 45 of 1,803 infants born to women using this drug (2.5 percent) had serious birth defects; this does not exceed the incidence of birth defects in the general population. **Possible adverse effects:** Ovarian hyperstimulation syndrome, enlarged ovaries, hot flushes, breast tenderness, gastric upset and, rarely, blood clots in the lung, ovarian cysts, uterine bleeding, hair loss, headache, dizziness.
METRODIN (Serono)	Urofollitropin (injection)	**How it works:** Stimulates ovarian follecular growth in women with polycystic ovarian disease (PCO) who failed to respond adequately to clomiphene citrate; follow-up treatment with human chorionic gonadotropin may be required to induce ovulation. **How well it succeeds:** In one clinical study of 189 PCO women, 88 percent ovulated after taking this drug and 30 percent became pregnant; 26 percent suffered a miscarriage. **Multiple births/birth defects:** 17 percent of the women treated with this drug had multiple fetuses. The incidence of birth defects among babies born to women who

Brand Name (Supplier)	Generic Name	Product Information
		took this drug does not exceed that found in the general population. **Possible adverse effects:** Blood clots in the lung, ovarian hyperstimulation syndrome, increased risk of ectopic pregnancy, ovarian cysts, enlarged ovary, abdominal pain, skin rashes, headache, breast tenderness
PERGONAL (Serono)	Menotropins (injection)	**How it works:** Menotropins contains gonadotropins from the urine of postmenopausal women. They stimulate follecular growth and maturation but do not cause ovulation, so they are coupled with human chorionic gonadotropin, which stimulates the release of the mature egg. **How well it succeeds:** Of 1,286 women who received menotropins, 75 percent ovulated and 25 percent became pregnant; 25 percent suffered a miscarriage. **Multiple births/birth defects:** 20 percent of the women who become pregnant while using this drug have multiple fetuses; 5 percent have 3 or more fetuses. In one study of 287 women who became pregnant and delivered babies after using this drug, 5 children were born with serious birth defects; these were not attributed to the drug. **Possible adverse effects:** Lung complications, including blood clots; ovarian hyperstimulation syndrome; ovarian cysts; enlarged ovaries; abdominal pain; skin rashes; dizziness

Brand Name (Supplier)	Generic Name	Product Information
PROFASI (Serono)	Chorionic gonadotropin (injection)	**How it works:** HCG is a hormone produced by the placenta. Like the pituitary hormones, LH and FSH, it stimulates the production and release of the egg from the ovary. It is used to treat women whose infertility is causes by a lack of these hormones. **How well it succeeds:** See menotropins, urofollitropin **Multiple births/birth defects:** See menotropins, urofollitropin **Possible adverse effects:** Headache, restlessness, fatigue, depression, swollen breasts, water retention
SEROPHANE (Serono)	see CLOMID	

Source: Physicians' Desk Reference, 48th ed. (Montvale, NJ: Medical Economics Data, 1994)

SOURCES

"Abortion pill to be tested in a new use," *New York Times,* May 4, 1994.

Adler, T., "Pill ups cancer risk in young women," *Science News,* June 10, 1995.

Advantage 24 professional advertising, *U.S. Pharmacist,* January 1995.

"Advisory committee on use of oral contraceptives in older women," Talk Paper, Food and Drug Administration, October 31, 1989.

Boston Women's Health Book Collective, *The New Our Bodies, Ourselves* (New York: Touchstone Books, 1992).

Bouchez, Colette, "Facing Reality," *[N.Y.] Daily News,* August 29, 1994.

Carrier, Roberta S., "Contraceptive methods and products," *Handbook of Nonprescription Drugs,* 9th ed. (Washington, DC: American Pharmaceutical Association, 1990).

"Condoms, contraceptives and STDs: Does your birth control method protect you from sexually transmitted disease?" (Research Triangle Park, NC: American Social Health Association, 1994).

"Deadly duo leads to cancer of the cervix," *Science News,* January 16, 1993.

Deveny, Kathleen, "Market grows fertile for pregnancy tests," *Wall Street Journal,* March 3, 1990.

Farr, Guston, et al., "Contraceptive efficacy and acceptability of the female condom," *American Journal of Public Health,* December 1994.

Fugh-Berman, Adriane, "Testimony of the National Women's Health Network before the [Food and Drug Administration] Fertility and Maternity Health Advisory Committee," October 26, 1989.

"Hormonal Contraception," *ACOG Technical Bulletin,* Number 198, October 1994 (Washington, DC: American College of Obstetricians and Gynecologists).

"How reliable are condoms?' *Consumer Reports,* May 1995.

Kolata, Gina, "Surveys find lack of knowledge limits use of morning-after pill," *New York Times,* March 29, 1995.

Kowblansky, Anna Charuk, "Overcoming infertility," *U.S. Pharmacist,* September 1994.

Krattenmaker, Tom, "Research finds female condom effective against

HIV transmission," *Princeton Weekly Bulletin,* April 11, 1994.

Krieger, John N., "New sexually transmitted disease treatment guidelines," *Journal of Urology,* July 1995.

"Norplant devices for birth control safe, F.D.A. says," *New York Times,* August 20, 1995.

"The Norplant system approved as new contraceptive implant," FDA Medical Bulletin, March 1991.

O'Connell, Mary Beth, "Vaginal dryness," *U.S. Pharmacist,* September 1994.

"Only manufacturer discontinues sponge for contraception," *New York Times,* January 11, 1995.

"Oral contraceptives, your patients, and daylight," Neutrogena Moisture SPF 15 Formula advertisement in *U.S. Pharmacist,* May 1995.

"Ortho releases 25th annual birth control study," press release, Ortho Pharmaceutical Corporation, October 12, 1993.

Package inserts for DEPO-PROVERA, REALITY, assorted male condoms.

"A pill for the 'morning after,'" September 19, 1994 (Washington, DC: American College of Obstetricians and Gynecologists).

Physicians' Desk Reference, 48th ed. (Montvale, NJ: Medical Economics Data, 1994).

Physicians' Desk Reference for Nonprescription Drugs, 16th ed. (Montvale, NJ: Medical Economics Data, 1995).

Raeburn, Paul, "The female condom," *Glamour,* February 1995.

Rinzler, Carol Ann, "The return of the condom," *American Health,* July 1987.

Ryder, R. E. J., "Natural family planning: Effective birth control supported by the Catholic Church," *British Medical Journal,* September 18, 1993.

Seaman, Barbara, *The Doctors' Case Against the Pill* (Alameda, CA: Hunter House, 1996).

Seaman, Barbara, and Gideon Seaman, M.D., *Women and the Crisis in Sex Hormones* (New York: Rawson Associates, 1977).

Simons, G. L., *Simons' Book of World Sexual Records* (New York: Pyramid Books, 1975).

"Study confirms it: Female condom works well," press release, Wisconsin Pharmacal, January 3, 1995.

Tanenbaum, Leora, "Pill politics," *Boston Phoenix,* February 24, 1995.

Trussell, James, et al., "Comparative contraceptive efficacy of the female condom and other barrier methods," *Family Planning Perspectives,* March/April 1994.

"Twenty-Third Ortho Annual Birth Control Study," Ortho Pharmaceutical Corporation, 1991.

"Unique contraceptive no longer available," *Consumer Reports,* September 1995.

"Urinary infections and spermicides," *New Woman,* April 1995.

Vaughn, Paul, *The Pill on Trial* (London: Weidenfeld and Nicolson, 1972).

Zamula, Evelyn, "New help for urinary tract infections," *FDA Consumer,* June 1995.

CHAPTER 4

VITAMINS AND MINERALS

For some of us, it started with cod liver oil; for others, it was the Flintstones, those funny little pills slipped onto the breakfast plate. Then came the multivitamin "just for insurance," an iron pill to fight anemia, extra vitamin C to protect against colds or stimulate immune function, and calcium to strengthen bones in preparation for the loss of bone density at menopause.

In the past decade, American medical research has expanded to include a hard investigation of nondrug therapeutic regimens, including nutrition. In the fall of 1993, the National Institutes of Health created the Office of Alternative Medicine specifically to fund controlled studies measuring the true effectiveness of therapies as various as biofeedback for diabetes, guided imagery for asthma, and hypnosis to speed healing of broken bones. The list also includes studies on nutritional supplements. Eventually, we will know whether changing our diet or upping our consumption of vitamins can prevent or cure disease or enhance the healing and preventive potential of many orthodox medical treatments.

WHAT ARE VITAMINS AND MINERALS?

Vitamins and minerals are chemical substances essential for life. Vitamins are organic, derived from living material. They occur naturally in plants and animals. There are two types of vitamins, those that dissolve in fat (fat soluble) and those that dissolve in water (water soluble).

Minerals are inorganic; they come from nonliving substances such as rocks and metals. There are two categories of minerals, the *major minerals,* which are present in amounts greater than 0.01 percent of the body's weight, and the *minor minerals,* which are present in even smaller amounts. As a rule, our dietary requirements for major minerals are greater than 100 mg a day, while our requirements for trace minerals are less than 100 mg a day.

Chemically speaking, there is absolutely no difference between the vitamins and minerals we get from food and those we get from supplements. It is true that supplements labeled "natural" or "organic" may omit artificial colors and flavors as well as sugar and starch fillers. This can be very important to someone who is allergic to one or another of these ingredients, but it has no effect on the potency of the product. In addition, some vitamins marked "natural" or "organic" may be supplemented with synthetic vitamins as well. For example, rose hips are a natural source of ascorbic acid (vitamin C), but the amount they provide is relatively small, so synthetic ascorbic acid is added to make it possible for the manufacturer to produce a tablet of an acceptable size.

In the end, vitamin C is vitamin C whether it comes from an orange or a pill. The difference between the two is that pills only supply the vitamin. The orange, however, is a package deal: energy (calories), plus a variety of others vitamins and minerals, some fiber, and best of all, something that tastes good. That's why supplements should always be used (as their name implies) in addition to food, not as a substitute for it.

FAT-SOLUBLE VITAMINS

VITAMIN A   (retinol) keeps skin supple and moistens mucous membranes—the tissues lining the eyes, nose, mouth, throat, vagina, and rectum. It protects night vision, bone growth, tooth development, and reproductive functions. Our bodies obtain vitamin A in one of two forms, either as *retinol* (preformed vitamin A) from animal foods such as liver (beef, calf, pork, chicken, and turkey), fish (salmon), or supplements, or by converting *carotenes* (vitamin A precursors) in plant foods to retinol.

VITAMIN D   enables the body to absorb calcium. The best source of vitamin D for Americans is fortified milk. Fish oils, such as cod liver oil, are a good source of vitamin D, which is also known as "the sunshine vitamin" because our own body fat contains steroid compounds that are converted to vitamin D when we are exposed to sunlight.

VITAMIN E   protects muscles, nerves, and the cardiovascular system. Recent studies show that high levels of vitamin E appear to prevent low density lipoproteins (LDLs), the fat and protein particles that carry cholesterol into arteries, from sticking to the artery walls and clogging the blood vessels. A 1995 study of healthy men at the University of Texas Southwestern Medical Center in Dallas found that 400 IU of vitamin E a day counters LDLs. Vitamin E also reduces blood clotting; one small study of people with blood vessel disease showed that daily doses of vitamin E plus aspirin were more effective against heart attack and stroke than aspirin alone. We get vitamin E from tocopherols and tocotrienols, two groups of chemical compounds in vegetable oils, nuts, and whole-grain cereals.

VITAMIN K   is a group of chemicals essential for the formation of prothrombin and several other proteins required for blood clotting. The best dietary source of this vitamin is green leafy vegetables; vitamin K is also produced by bacteria living normally in our intestinal tract.

WATER-SOLUBLE VITAMINS

VITAMIN C   (ascorbic acid) plays an important role in developing and maintaining connective tissue. It prevents scurvy, the deficiency disease whose symptoms include slow wound healing, bleeding gums leading to tooth loss, easy bruising, muscle pains, and skin rashes. The best sources of vitamin C are citrus fruits. Other fruits and vegetables such as broccoli, brussels sprouts, cabbage, cantaloupe, fresh peppers, snow peas, strawberries, sweet potatoes, and tomatoes also provide respectable amounts.

THIAMIN (VITAMIN B1)   protects the heart and nervous system. The thiamin deficiency disease, beriberi, causes nerve inflammation, irregular heartbeat, enlarged heart, loss of muscle tissue, and mental confusion.

RIBOFLAVIN (VITAMIN B2)   is essential for many enzyme reactions and enables body cells to use oxygen to release energy from the foods we eat. It works in tandem with vitamin B6 and niacin. A diet deficient in riboflavin may lead to dermatitis, inflammation of mucous membranes, and a form of anemia. Dietary sources of riboflavin include meat, fish, milk, eggs, and liver.

NIACIN (NICOTINIC ACID, NICOTINAMIDE)   is an essential element in many enzyme reactions, vital processes including the metabolism of sugars and fats and the oxygenation of body cells. The niacin deficiency disease, pellagra, is characterized by diarrhea, inflammation of the skin and mucous membranes, and, in severe cases, dementia. Meat is the best source of preformed niacin. It also contains tryptophan, an amino acid that is converted to niacin in the body. For comparison purposes, 60 mg tryptophan = 1 mg niacin = 1 niacin equivalent (NE).

VITAMIN B6   includes three related chemicals, pyridoxine, pyridoxal, and pyridoxamine. In the liver, they are converted to pyridoxal phosphate and pyridoxamine phosphate, which are required for the metabolism of fats and amino acids, the building blocks of proteins. The richest sources of this vitamin are liver, chicken, fish, pork, lamb, milk, eggs, unmilled rice, soy beans, whole wheat products, peanuts, and walnuts.

FOLATE (FOLACIN, FOLIC ACID)   carries carbon molecules from one compound to another during the metabolism and synthesis of proteins. In 1995, researchers discovered that folate appears to reduce the risk of heart attack by lowering blood levels of the amino acid homocysteine, which is converted to an amino acid that stimulates brain cell receptors at normal levels but causes cells to self-destruct at excess levels.

VITAMIN B12   is unique, in that it is the only vitamin that contains a mineral (cobalt). This nutrient maintains the myelin covering of the nerves, spinal cord, and brain; a deficiency may lead to neurological and psychiatric disorders. There is no vitamin B12 in plant foods. We get what we need from foods of animal origin: meat, fish, poultry, eggs, milk, cheese, and yogurt. In addition, the bacteria living in our intestinal tract manufacture small amounts of vitamin B12.

PANTOTHENIC ACID   is a B-vitamin that plays a role in a wide variety of enzyme actions such as the release of energy from carbohydrates and the synthesis of fatty acids and steroid hormones. It is widely available in foods, especially meat, fish, poultry, whole grain cereals, and beans.

BIOTIN   enables our bodies to synthesize proteins from amino acids. It is found in whole grains, eggs, peanuts, oysters, and liver.

CHOLINE   is essential for the metabolism of fats. It comes from whole grains, liver, seeds, and green leafy vegetables.

PANTOTHENIC ACID   (which sometimes appears on labels as calcium pantothenate) helps us extract energy from carbohydrates and synthesize fatty acids and steroid hormones.

MAJOR MINERALS

CALCIUM   makes strong bones and teeth and protects our muscles, preventing them from going into spasm. The best sources of calcium are milk and other dairy products, as well as certain vegetables such as broccoli and kale.

PHOSPHOROUS   acts in concert with calcium and is an essential component of bone. It is so widely distributed in foods that deficiency is rare.

MAGNESIUM   is required for all biosynthesis in the body, including the transfer of materials across cell membranes, the transmission of nerve impulses, and the transmission of genetic codes. Like phosphorus, magnesium is widely available in foods, with the highest concentrations found in whole seeds (nuts, beans, grains) and bananas.

TRACE ELEMENTS

IRON   is essential to the production of hemoglobin, the pigment in red blood cells that carries oxygen throughout the body. There are respectable amounts of iron in organ meats (liver, heart, kidneys), egg yolks, wheat germ, and oysters.

ZINC   is a component of the enzymes involved in most major metabolic body functions and a major influence on male reproductive function. We get zinc from meat, liver, eggs, and seafood, especially oysters. Grains are also rich in zinc, but fiber and other chemicals in plants interfere with our body's ability to absorb the zinc.

IODINE   is a component of the thyroid hormones thyroxin and triiodothyronine. An iodine deficiency may cause goiter (a swollen thyroid gland) or cretinism (a form of mental and physical retardation). Iodine occurs naturally in seafood and food grown near the ocean.

VITAMINS

Fat Soluble	Water Soluble
Vitamin A	Vitamin C
Vitamin D	Thiamin (vitamin B1)
Vitamin E	Riboflavin (vitamin B2)
Vitamin K	Folate
	Niacin
	Vitamin B6 (pyridoxine)
	Vitamin B12 (cyanocobalamin)
	Pantothenic acid

MINERALS

Major Minerals	Trace Elements
Calcium	Iron
Phosphorus	Zinc
Magnesium	Iodine
Sodium*	Selenium
Potassium*	Copper
Chlorine*	Manganese
Sulfur	Fluoride
	Molybdenum

* These are also commonly known as *electrolytes,* substances that regulate the body's fluid balance.

RECOMMENDED DIETARY ALLOWANCES

The recommended dietary allowances (RDAs), set by the National Research Council's Food and Nutrition Board, are safe, effective doses of vitamins and minerals for boys and girls, men and women in specific age groups. A less comprehensive set of values, known as the U.S. Recommended Daily Allowances (U.S. RDAs), based on the Recommended Dietary Allowances published in 1968, is still used for labeling on vitamin and mineral products. The U.S. RDAs are daily recommendations for broad groups of people, i.e., "adults," rather than people aged 19 to 24, 25 to 29, and so forth.

The first RDAs were issued in 1941 by the National Research Council's Committee on Food and Nutrition (now the Food and Nutrition Board), set up in 1940 to advise on "nutritional problems in connection with the National Defense." Right from the start, the RDAs were generous, providing a "margin of safety" for healthy people. They were also designed to make it easy for homemakers to plan several days' menus at once. The RDAs are an average of what you should consume daily over several days. The "D" in RDA stands for *dietary,* not *daily.*

Through eight revisions over more than 40 years, the RDAs sailed along with no major policy disagreements to ruffle the waters. That changed in 1985 when the National Research Council Food and Nutrition Board Committee, working on the ninth revision, proposed lowering the RDAs for several nutrients, including vitamins A and C.

The committee wanted to raise the RDA for vitamin C for smokers (who seem to metabolize this nutrient more quickly) and lower it for adult nonsmokers. They also wanted to lower the RDA for vitamin A for everybody.

But by 1985, statisticians had begun to accumulate evidence suggesting that specific foods and nutrients really might play a role in preventing or treating some chronic diseases. Most exciting was the growing body of epidemiological data to suggest that vitamin C and foods rich in carotenoids, the red and yellow vitamin A precursors in fruits and vegetables, might lower the risk of some cancers. Neither proposal, therefore, was publicly acceptable.

There were also political problems. The RDAs are more than handy guidelines for planning home menus. They are also the numbers used to plan menus for nutrition programs such as school lunches and Meals-on-Wheels. Because the RDA report is funded by the National Institutes of Health and the United States Public Health Service, lowering the RDAs could be construed as providing scientific justification for cutting government-funded nutritional programs, an aim of the Reagan White House in the mid-1980s and the Republican-controlled Congress in the mid-1990s.

As a result, in the summer of 1985, the Food and Nutrition Board turned the report down flat, and the National Research Council announced that new RDAs would not be released in 1985. The committee was disbanded, and a second one was set up. Its report, the tenth edition of the recommended dietary allowances, appeared in the fall of 1989 with no reductions in the RDAs for vitamins A and C and higher RDAs for smokers.

A number of controversies, however, remain unresolved.

First, the RDA for iron for women of childbearing age was lowered from 18 mg to 15 mg. The scientists cited new research suggesting that we absorb iron more efficiently than previously assumed and can get by on less. Whether the lower RDA will protect menstruating women from iron-deficiency anemia remains to be seen.

Second, the RDA for calcium rose from 800 mg to 1,200 mg for young men and women aged 19 to 24, but the RDA for adults older than 25 stayed at 800 mg. These guidelines ignore a 1984 National Institutes of Health Conference advisory to set the RDA for healthy women of childbearing age at 1,000 mg and the RDA for post-menopausal women at 1,000 mg for those taking estrogen and 1,500 mg for those not using hormone replacement therapy. (These recommendations were confirmed in a 1994 NIH Consensus Statement on optimal calcium intake.)

Third, despite recent studies showing that older people may need larger amounts of vitamin B12 (which helps prevent anemia) and vitamin B6 (needed to synthesize proteins), the RDAs for these two nutrients were lowered. This prompted the American Association of Retired People, among others, to advise the elderly to ignore the new RDAs in favor of the recommendations of a 1989 National Research Council report, "Diet and Health: Implications for Reducing Chronic Disease Risk," which called for higher amounts of some nutrients than the new RDA report. As of this writing, the 1989 RDAs remain the latest official guidelines on recommended dietary allowances.

Most of the RDAs in the following tables of RDAs for women and pregnant or nursing women are shown in milligrams (mg) and micrograms (mcg). There are special descriptions for three nutrients, vitamins A, D, and E.

The RDA for vitamin A is listed in units "retinol equivalents" (mcg RE), that is, the amount needed to match one microgram of the "pre-formed" vitamin A derived from foods of animal origin such as liver.

Vitamin D is actually three compounds: vitamin D1 (lumisterol plus ergocalciferol), vitamin D2 (ergocalciferol), and vitamin D3 (cholecalciferol). The RDA for vitamin D is measured in equivalents of cholecalciferol: 10 mcg of cholecalciferol = 400 IU of vitamin D.

The compund with the greatest vitamin E activity is alpha-tocopherol. If you rate this one at 100, the relative vitamin E activity values of beta-tocopherol is 25–50; of gamma-tocopherol, 10–35; and of alpha-tocotrienol, 30. The RDA for vitamin E is measured in milligrams of alpha-tocopherol equivalents (mg a-TE).

RDAS FOR WOMEN

Nutrient	Unit	Age Group				
		11–14	15–18	19–24	25–50	51+
Vitamin A	mcg RE IU*	800 4,000	800 4,000	800 4,000	800 4,000	800 4,000
Vitamin D	mcg IU*	10 400	10 400	10 400	10 400	10 400
Vitamin E	mg a-TE IU*	8 30	8 30	8 30	8 30	8 30
Vitamin K	mcg	45	55	60	65	65
Vitamin C	mg	60	60	60	60	60
Thiamin (vitamin B1)	mg	1.1	1.1	1.1	1.1	1.0
Riboflavin (vitamin B2)	mg	1.3	1.3	1.3	1.3	1.2
Niacin	mg	15	15	15	15	13
Vitamin B6	mg	1.4	1.5	1.6	1.6	1.6
Folate	mcg	150	150	150	150	180
Vitamin B12 (cyanocobalamin)	mcg	2	2	2	2	2
Calcium	mg	1,200	1,200	1,200	800	800
Phosphorus	mg	1,200	1,200	1,200	800	800
Magnesium	mg	280	300	280	280	280
Iron	mg	15	15	15	15	10
Zinc	mg	12	12	12	12	12
Iodine	mcg	150	150	150	150	150

* Values listed in IUs are U.S. RDAs used for labeling on vitamin and mineral products.

Source: National Research Council, Recommended Dietary Allowances, 10th ed. (Washington, DC: National Academy Press, 1989).

RDAS FOR PREGNANT OR NURSING WOMEN

Nutrient	Unit	Pregnant	Nursing: First 6 mo.	Nursing: Second 6 mo.
Vitamin A	mcg RE IU*	800	1,300	1,200
Vitamin D	mcg IU*	10	10	10
Vitamin E	mg a-TE IU*	10	12	11
Vitamin K	mcg	65	65	65
Vitamin C	mg	75	95	90
Thiamin (vitamin B1)	mg	1.5	1.6	1.6
Riboflavin (vitamin B2)	mg	1.6	1.8	1.7
Niacin	mg	17	20	20
Vitamin B6	mg	2.2	2.6	2.6
Folate	mcg	400	280	260
Vitamin B12 (cyanocobalamin)	mcg	2.2	2.6	2.6
Calcium	mg	1,200	1,200	1,200
Phosphorus	mg	1,200	1,200	1,200
Magnesium	mg	320	355	340
Iron	mg	30	15	15
Zinc	mg	15	19	16
Iodine	mcg	175	200	200

Values listed in IUs are U.S. RDAs used for labeling on vitamin and mineral products.

Source: National Research Council, *Recommended Dietary Allowances,* 10th ed. (Washington, DC: National Academy Press, 1989).

MEGADOSES

RDAs are protective, not therapeutic. They are assumed to prevent a deficiency, but they may not cure an existing one, so a lot of people naturally wonder whether they should be taking larger doses on a daily basis.

Very large amounts of vitamins and minerals are known colloquially as megadoses. Megadoses may be several hundred times the RDA. In some cases, they appear to be harmless or even useful. In others, they are potentially dangerous.

FAT-SOLUBLE VITAMINS   Megadoses of vitamins A, D, and E are troublesome because excess amounts of these vitamins are stored in body fat rather than excreted. In adults, the continued use of very high doses of retinol (25,000 IU or more) may lead to liver damage, pressure inside the skull, headache, vomiting, vision problems, hair loss, loss of appetite, dryness of the mucous membranes, cracked lips, joint and bone pain, low-grade fever, and itching. Very large doses of carotenoids may temporarily turn skin orange but do not appear to be toxic.

The toxic doses of vitamin D may be as low as five times the RDA. Symptoms of vitamin D poisoning include heightened levels of calcium in blood and urine that may lead to calcium deposits in soft tissue that can cause irreversible kidney and heart damage.

Vitamin E is relatively nontoxic in amounts as high as 100 times the RDA. Given the recent evidence of vitamin E's ability to protect against heart and vascular disease, a 1993 study from the USDA Beltsville Nutrition Research Center suggests that raising the RDA for vitamin E in multivitamin products may turn out to be the most effective way to increase consumption of this nutrient. The study, run by researchers from the National Cancer Institute and the Agricultural Research Service, compared plasma levels of vitamin E in three groups of volunteers: those who took no vitamin supplements, those who got an extra 15 to 60 IU from a daily multivitamin, and those who took a 100 IU vitamin E capsule each day. The group taking multivitamin supplements fared best: their blood levels of vitamin E were 14 percent higher than those of the group that took no vitamins and more than twice as high as those who took plain vitamin E capsules.

Even over long periods of time, large amounts of vitamin K do not appear to be harmful to healthy people. However, vitamin K may reduce the effectiveness of anticoagulants (COUMARIN, WARFARIN).

WATER-SOLUBLE VITAMINS   Despite early warnings that mega-doses of vitamin C might lead to the formation of kidney stones, the effects of very large amounts of vitamin C have turned out to be rela-tively benign: upset stomach, constipation, or diarrhea. As for the benefits, research has shown that large doses of the vitamin reduce symptoms and may cut the duration of a cold by a fraction of a day. More recent studies of vitamin C megadoses suggest that they may raise blood levels of HDLs, the "good" fat and protein particles that carry cholesterol and fat out of the body. In 1995, an eight-month study of 138 male and female volunteers from the USDA Human Nu-trition Research Center on Aging at Tufts University in Boston showed that a 1-gram (1,000 mg) vitamin C supplement each day raised the levels of HDL cholesterol 8 percent for people with blood levels of vitamin C lower than 1 milligram per deciliter (mg/dl) but had no effect on people with higher blood levels.

Some B vitamins appear to be virtually nontoxic even in very high doses. Oral megadoses of thiamin (vitamin B1) are readily ex-creted in urine; doses as high as 500 times the RDA taken once a day for a month have produced no ill effects. There has never been a re-ported incidence of toxicity from riboflavin (vitamin B2). The RDA for vitamin B12 (cyanocobalamin) for healthy adults is 1 microgram; there is no evidence of toxicity at up to 100 times this amount.

On the other hand, megadoses (100 to 1,000 mg per day) of nicotinic acid may cause liver damage as well as blood vessel dilation (flushing). Niacinamide is less likely to cause flushing.

Most healthy adults can consume as much as 10 times the RDA for vitamin B6 (pyridoxine) with no apparent ill effects, but very large doses (1,000 mg or more) over long periods of time may cause severe peripheral neuropathies—damage to nerves in hands, feet, arms, and legs. The damage and resultant pain is usually slowly reversible when the megadoses cease.

Megadoses of folate (starting at 100 times the RDA) may trigger convulsions in people with epilepsy whose seizures are controlled by the drug phenytoin, but there is virtually no data regarding toxicity in otherwise healthy people. Nonetheless, excessive amounts are not rec-ommended.

MAJOR MINERALS

The 1989 RDAs set calcium levels very low (only 800 mg for women older than 24). Current recommendations are 1,000 mg a day for pre-menopausal women and 1,500 mg a day for postmenopausal women who are not using estrogen. There are no reports of adverse effects among people taking as much 1,500 mg a day, but higher doses can prove troublesome. Constipation is a common side effect among healthy people taking 1,500 to 4,000 mg calcium a day, and this much calcium may inhibit the body's absorption of iron, zinc, and other minerals. People whose bodies do not absorb calcium well may suffer kidney damage caused by high levels of calcium circulating in the blood. These effects may occur in everyone who takes more than 4,000 mg calcium a day. The most common cause of calcium toxicity is consuming large amounts of antacids.

Consuming very large amounts of phosphorus reduces the level of calcium in the blood. Large doses of magnesium do not seem to be harmful to people with normal kidney function. People with kidney disease, however, may develop irregular heartbeat and respiratory problems that, left untreated, may be fatal.

TRACE ELEMENTS   All trace elements are toxic when consumed in excessive amounts. For example, in children, three grams (3,000 mg) of iron may be lethal; for adults, the lethal dose starts at 200 mg for each kilogram (2.2 pounds) of body weight.

Zinc poisoning (gastric irritation and vomiting) may follow megadoses of 2 grams zinc. Smaller amounts, in the range of 18.5 to 25 mg a day, may interfere with the body's ability to use copper; taking 300 mg a day (20 times the RDA for healthy adult women) for 6 weeks has been shown to inhibit immune function. In addition, excess zinc may raise cholesterol levels, increasing the risk of heart disease.

Copper is poisonous in large amounts, as, for example, what one might find in an acidic food cooked in an unlined copper pot. Inhaled as dust, manganese is a neurotoxin. Chromium seems to be safe in laboratory animals given as much as 100 mg per kilogram (2.2 pounds) of body weight. Large amounts of molybdenum (10 to 15 mg per day) inhibit copper metabolism and may cause a goutlike condition. Very small amounts of fluoride in drinking water strengthen tooth enamel, but large amounts, sometimes from naturally fluoridated well water, cause fluorosis, a syndrome characterized by fatigue, weakness, brittle bones, and mottled teeth.

ESTIMATED SAFE AND ADEQUATE
DAILY DIETARY INTAKE*

Nutrient	Unit	Age Group				
		11–14	15–18	19–24	25–50	51+
Biotin	mcg	30–100	30–100	30–100	30–100	30–100
Choline	no RDA set					
Pantothenic Acid	mg	4–7	4–7	4–7	4–7	4–7
Copper	mg	1.5–2.5	1.5–3	1.5–3	1.5–3	1.5–3
Manganese	mg	2–5	2–5	2–5	2–5	2–5
Fluoride	mg	1.5–2.5	1.5–4	1.5–4	1.5–4	1.5–4
Chromium	mcg	50–200	50–200	50–200	50–200	50–200
Molybdenum	mcg	75–250	75–250	75–250	75–250	75–250

There is not enough information on the nutrients in this chart to create RDAs. However, the National Research Council, which sets RDAs, has recommended the "safe and adequate" daily dietary intake levels given here.

Source: National Research Council, *Recommended Dietary Allowances,* 10th ed. (Washington, DC: National Academy Press, 1989).

NUTRIENT/DRUG INTERACTIONS

One unexpected side effect of vitamins and minerals is their interaction with various drugs. The tables on pages 133–134 list many of the more common nutrient/drug interactions. *Note: this is not a comprehensive list of all possible interactions. As nutritional research expands, it is likely that there will be additions to this guide. Always seek your doctor's advice on nutritional requirements when you are taking medicine before adding or subtracting nutrients or supplements from your diet.*

A SELECTED LIST OF VITAMIN, MINERAL, AND DRUG INTERACTIONS

This drug	...and these nutrients	...interact in this manner
Aspirin	vitamin C, thiamine, folic acid	aspirin increases excretion of these vitamins in urine
	iron	chronic use of aspirin irritates stomach lining, causing blood loss that may result in iron deficiency
Barbiturates	vitamin C	barbiturates increase the body's requirement for vitamin C; people who do not get RDA amounts may develop deficiency
Cholestyramine (anticholesterol)	vitamins A, D, E, K	this drug alters absorption of fats and may lead to deficiency of fat-soluble vitamins
	folic acid, vitamin B12	possible vitamin deficiency
Cimetidine (anticholesterol)	iron	this drug reduces the body's absorption of iron
Clofibrate (anticholesterol)	folic acid, vitamin B12, iron	possible vitamin deficiency
Colestipol (anticholesterol)	folic acid	possible vitamin deficiency
Corticosteroids	calcium	corticosteroids reduce the body's absorption of calcium
	vitamin C, vitamin B6, calcium, zinc	corticosteroids increase excretion or use of these nutrients leading to possible deficiency
Diuretics	calcium, potassium, magnesium, zinc	increased loss of minerals through urination may lead to deficiencies

This drug	...and these nutrients	...interact in this manner
Fenfluamine	vitamins A, D, E, K	may impair absorption of fats and fat-soluble vitamins
Laxatives containing mineral oil, biscodyl, diphenyl-methane, phenophthalein	vitamins A, D, E, K calcium, potassium	if used frequently or for long periods of time, laxatives lower the body's absorption of these vitamins
Indomethacin	iron	chronic use of indomethacin irritates stomach lining, causes blood loss that may result in iron deficiency
Penicillin	vitamin K, folic acid, vitamin B6, vitamin B12, calcium, magnesium	penicillin decreases absorption of or inactivates these nutrients
Sulfasalazine, sulfisoxazole, sulfamethaoxazole	folic acid	these drugs reduce the body's ability to absorb folic acid
Tetracyclines	calcium, magnesium, iron, zinc	normal amounts of these minerals in dairy foods bind and inactivate tetracyclines, reducing the antibiotics' effectiveness; this reaction also reduces the amounts of the minerals available to the body

Sources: James W. Long and James J. Rybacki, *The Essential Guide to Prescription Drugs* (New York: HarperCollins, 1994). Brian L. G. Morgan, *The Food and Drug Interaction Guide* (New York: Simon and Schuster, 1986). *Physicians' Desk Reference*, 48th ed. (Montvale, NJ: Medical Economics Data, 1994).

VITAMINS, MINERALS, AND REPRODUCTION

Vitamins and minerals play an essential role in maintaining healthy reproductive organs and ensuring that our reproductive systems function smoothly.

MENSTRUATION

Thiamine (vitamin B1) is a mild diuretic that may offer some relief for women who feel bloated in the days before menstrual bleeding begins. Vitamin B6 (pyridoxine) is sometimes credited with easing menstrual discomfort, but the evidence is mostly anecdotal. No significant clinical benefits have been consistently demonstrated. At the same time, large doses of vitamin B6 may cause nerve damage serious enough to interfere with walking. In one study, four of seven women taking gram quantities (doses in multiples of 1,000 mg) were severely disabled; similar symptoms have been reported in women taking as little as 50 mg a day.

Most women of childbearing age are deficient in iron because their diets do not provide enough to make up for what is lost during the menstrual flow. On average, a woman loses 60 to 80 ml of blood each month, representing about 1.4 mg iron. Some women, however, may lose as much as 100 to 200 ml of blood, with a consequent greater loss of iron. Because it is virtually impossible to get all the iron you need from the customary 1,500- to 2,000-calorie-a-day American diet, the usual remedy is an iron supplement.

Vitamin C is a valuable aid because it increases the body's absorption of iron. Consuming 25 to 75 mg of vitamin C a day, in food or supplements, can double or quadruple the amount of iron absorbed through the intestines. Vitamin C supplements even increase the amount of iron absorbed from plant foods, traditionally an inefficient way to get iron. Iron deficiency reduces levels of the active thyroid hormone, T3. But a 1992 ten-week USDA–Grand Forks Human Nutrition Research study of women on a low-meat diet showed that taking a 500-mg vitamin C tablet with each meal significantly boosted their T3 levels.

CONTRACEPTION

To date, the National Research Council has not created specific RDAs for women using either birth control pills or an IUD, but it is clear that oral contraceptives interact with a number of nutrients.

For example, the long-term, daily use of vitamin C megadoses (1,000 mg or more) increases blood levels of estrogen from the pill. Birth control pills decrease the body's ability to absorb thiamin (vitamin B1), riboflavin (vitamin B2), and folate, and the ability of vitamin B6 to metabolize the amino acid tryptophan is reduced by estrogens. Women using estrogen/progestin birth control pills may need vitamin B6 supplements.

Women who use an IUD may require iron supplements because the device irritates the lining of the uterus, producing a small but steady loss of blood.

PREGNANCY

Ordinarily, whether we choose to take vitamin and mineral supplements is a personal matter. But a pregnant woman's choices also affect her growing fetus. If she does not get sufficient amounts of certain nutrients, such as vitamin C, the baby may be born deficient. If she takes megadoses, the excess may cross the placenta. In very high doses, some vitamins, such as vitamin A, are teratogens, substances that cause birth defects. Others, such as folates, prevent damage to the fetus.

In general, the RDAs for vitamins and minerals are increased during pregnancy (see page 127). For information about the effects of deficiency or megadoses of vitamins or minerals during pregnancy, see the tables on pages 137–140.

LACTATION

The RDAs for a nursing mother have an extra margin of nutritional "insurance" to protect the infant. As in pregnancy, there is an intimate relationship between the mother's diet and her child's. Some of the effects of vitamins and minerals on women who are nursing are laid out in the tables on pages 141–142.

SOME EFFECTS OF DEFICIENCY OR MEGADOSES OF SELECTED VITAMINS AND MINERALS DURING PREGNANCY

Nutrient	RDA for Pregnant Women	Deficiencies/Megadoses
Vitamin A	1,000 mcg RE	**Megadoses:** Large amounts of vitamin A cross the placenta and are potentially teratogenic. Pregnant laboratory rats given doses of vitamin A 50 to 100 times their normal dietary requirement gave birth to deformed fetuses.
Vitamin D	10 mcg	**Deficiency:** Pregnant women and their fetuses need vitamin D in order to absorb calcium into bones. If the mother does not take in enough vitamin D, the fetus will take its calcium directly from the mother's bones. **Megadoses:** Large doses of vitamin D cross the placenta. In laboratory animals this led to fetal abnormalities.
Vitamin E	10 mg a-Te	**Deficiency:** The amount of tocopherol in a woman's blood rises during pregnancy along with the level of fats. A pregnant woman needs a slight increase in vitamin E to accomodate the growth of the fetus.
Vitamin K	65 mcg	**Megadoses:** If a pregnant women takes large amounts of vitamin K, her baby may be born jaundiced.
Vitamin C	70 mg	**Deficiency:** A pregnant woman's blood levels of vitamin C decrease while her fetus' blood levels rise; vitamin C is transported across the placenta to the child. A maternal deficiency, therefore, means a fetal deficicency. Women who smoke while pregnant have reduced levels of vitamin C, and the vitamin's transport to the fetus seems to be impaired—fetuses of smoking mothers get comparatively less vitamin C even when the mothers' blood levels are similar to those of nonsmokers.

Nutrient	RDA for Pregnant Women	Deficiencies/Megadoses
Vitamin C (cont'd)		**Megadoses:** Large amounts of vitamin C cross the placenta to saturate the body tissues of the developing fetus. A woman who takes megadoses of vitamin C while pregnant may give birth to a child who temporarily requires greater-than-normal doses simply to prevent deficiency. Eventually, the baby's requirement will return to normal.
Thiamin (vitamin B1)	1.5 mg	**Deficiency:** A pregnant woman whose diet lacks adequate vitamin B may develop the defiency disease beriberi, as will her fetus.
Riboflavin (vitamin B2)	1.6 mg	**Deficiency:** The increased growth and tissue synthesis in mother and fetus requires additional riboflavin; riboflavin-deficient laboratory animals produce offspring with a wide variety of abnormalities ranging from cleft palate to heart defects. If you are getting sufficient amounts of other vitamins, it is unlikely that you will have a riboflavin deficiency.
Niacin	17 mg	No effects reported.
Vitamin B6 (pyridoxine)	2.2 mg	**Deficiency:** Estrogens inhibit vitamin B6 metabolism of the amino acid tryptophan. High estrogen levels during pregnancy require supplementation to prevent deficiency. Some studies have suggested that infants born to women who take large doses of vitamin B6 while pregnant may be born dependent on this nutrient, temporarily requiring greater-than-normal amounts. (See Vitamin C as well.)

Nutrient	RDA for Pregnant Women	Deficiencies/Megadoses
Folate	400 mcg	**Deficiency:** Pregnant women whose diets do not contain sufficient amounts of folate have an increased risk of giving birth to a child with a neural tube (spinal tube) defect such as spina bifida, which currently occurs in 1 to 2 of every 1,000 babies born each year in the U.S. (4,000 children a year). Taking a folic acid supplement throughout pregnancy significantly reduces the risk of this birth defect.
Vitamin B12 (cyano-cobalamin)	2.2 mcg	No effects reported.
Calcium	1,200 mg	**Deficiency:** If a pregnant woman's diet does not contain enough calcium to sustain the growth of fetal bones, the fetus will draw calcium directly from the mother's bones. There is no guarantee that this provides enough calcium to produce strong, dense fetal bone tissue. **Megadoses:** Very large amounts of calcium reduce the absorption of zinc (see Zinc below).
Iron	30 mg	**Deficiency:** A pregnant woman needs enough iron to produce new blood for her own increased body tissues as well as for the placenta and fetus. If she does not get enough iron, she will not be able to manufacture sufficient hemoglobin for this "extra" blood, and the baby as well as the mother may become anemic. In the first few months of pregnancy, because she is no longer losing blood through menstruation, a woman probably does not need supplementation above the RDA for women who are not pregnant. Later in pregnancy, however, her increased requirements cannot be met by diet; they require a supplement.

Nutrient	RDA for Pregnant Women	Deficiencies/Megadoses
Zinc	15 mg	**Deficiency:** If a pregnant woman is zinc deficient, her fetus will be too. In pregnant animals, a zinc deficiency in the mother leads to a high incidence of fetal death or stillbirth and/or birth defects in virtually all organ systems. This has not been reported in human pregnancies. Data from a 1995, 580-woman study at the University of Alabama-Birmingham suggest that some women, especially thin women, will deliver bigger, healthier babies if they take 25-mg zinc supplements. Comparing 294 women who took the supplements with 286 who were given placebos, researchers found that babies born to the zinc group weighed an average of 4.5 oz more at birth. On average, their head circumference was 0.2 inch larger. The greatest improvement was among thin women. For example, women standing 5'4" tall and weighing 110 lbs had babies averaging 15 oz more if they took the supplements.

Sources: The Merck Manual, 16th ed. (Rahway, NJ: Merck Rsearch Laboratories, 1992). National Research Council, Recommended Dietary Allowances, 10th ed. (Washington, DC: National Academy Press, 1989). Jean D. Wilson, et al., eds., Harrison's Principles of Internal Medicine, 12th ed. (New York: McGraw Hill, 1991).

SOME EFFECTS OF SELECTED VITAMINS AND MINERALS WHILE NURSING

Nutrient	RDA for Nursing Mothers First 6 mo. (Second 6 mo.)	Effects
Vitamin A	1,300 mcg RE (1,200 mcg RE)	Women whose diets are low in vitamin A may require supplements to make up for the nutrient excreted in breast milk.
Vitamin D	10 mcg (10 mcg)	The RDA for nursing mothers is higher to make up for what is excreted in breast milk. Very large doses may be toxic to mother and child.
Vitamin E	12 mg a-TE IU* (11 mg a-TE IU)	Like the RDAs for vitamins A and D, the RDA for vitamin E is increased to make up for what is excreted in breast milk. Human milk has enough vitamin E to satisfy the infant's needs.
Vitamin K	65 mcg (65 mcg)	No reports of ill effects from taking more or less than the RDA.
Vitamin C	95 mg (90 mg)	A nursing woman loses about 18–22 mg a day in milk production. Daily increase of 35 mg satisfies the increased requirement.
Thiamin (vitamin B1)	1.6 mg (1.6 mg)	The thiamin-deficiency disease beriberi has been identified in babies breastfed by thiamin-deficient mothers. The disease, usually diagnosed in the second to fourth month of life, may cause weakness, "silent crying," paralysis, and heart failure. It is fatal if untreated.
Riboflavin (vitamin B2)	1.8 mg (1.7 mg)	No reports of ill effects from taking more or less than the RDA.
Niacin	20 mg (20 mg)	No reports of ill effects from taking more or less than the RDA.
Vitamin B6 (pyridoxine)	2.1 mg (2.1 mg)	No reports of ill effects from taking more or less than the RDA.

Nutrient	RDA for Nursing Mothers First 6 mo. (Second 6 mo.)	Effects
Folate	280 mcg (260 mcg)	Folic acid deficiency has been found in breastfed infants whose mothers were taking estrogen/progestin birth control pills while nursing.
Vitamin B12 (cyano-cobalamin)	2.6 mcg (2.6 mcg)	Signs of B12 deficiency have been seen in breastfed infants of women on strict vegan (no animal foods, no dairy products) diets.
Calcium	1,200 mg (1,200 mg)	If a nursing women does not get enough calcium, her body may draw from her bones to make her milk nutritious.
Phosphorus	1,200 mg (1,200 mg)	No reports of ill effects from taking more or less than the RDA.
Magnesium	355 mg (340 mg)	No reports of ill effects from taking more or less than the RDA.
Iron	15 mg (15 mg)	A woman loses less iron while nursing (about 0.15 to 0.3 mg a day) than during a menstrual period.
Zinc	19 mg (16 mg)	No reports of ill effects from taking more or less than the RDA.
Iodine	200 mcg (200 mcg)	No reports of ill effects from taking more or less than the RDA.
Selenium	75 mcg (75 mcg)	No reports of ill effects from taking more or less than the RDA.

Values listed in IUs are U.S. RDAs used for labeling on vitamin and mineral products.

Sources: *The Merck Manual,* 16th ed. (Rahway, NJ: Merck Research Laboratories., 1992). National Research Council, *Recommended Dietary Allowances,* 10th ed. (Washington, DC: National Academy Press, 1989). Jean D. Wilson, et al., eds., *Harrison's Principles of Internal Medicine,* 12th ed. (New York: McGraw Hill, 1991).

MENOPAUSE

Unfortunately, most information about vitamins and minerals for older women is anecdotal ("I tried this while I was going through menopause and discovered that . . .") rather than study-based. Although it appears that older women, like older men, may have nutrient requirements different from those of younger people, the RDAs issued in 1989 still consider all people older than 51 as a single age group. Therefore, hard facts about vitamins and minerals at menopause are hard to come by. When looking for advice, what we are likely to come up with is a lot of "maybes" such as these:

- Because vitamin A keeps skin and mucous membranes supple, it may be useful in protecting vaginal tissues as they thin and dry at menopause.

- A 1945 study reported in the *American Journal of Obstetrics and Gynecology* suggested that vitamin E supplements could help relieve hot flashes and drying tissues. Four years later, in a study of 66 women, half said their flashes and dry skin improved when they took 20 to 100 IU vitamin E a day. Since then, we've learned that vitamin E can protect the heart, but its effects on skin and hot flashes are still unproven.

What we know for sure is that at menopause, women begin to lose bone density very quickly. At one time, researchers believed that our bodies did not absorb calcium and build bone density after our middle twenties. Today, although it is still considered vital to accumulate bone while we are young, scientists have come to understand that increasing and maintaining calcium consumption as we grow older reduces the age-related loss of bone that leads to osteoporosis. This is particularly important for women who do not wish to take hormone replacement therapy.

As for heart disease, the major killer of older women, the news that the B vitamin folate (folic acid, folacin) may reduce the risk of heart attack by lowering blood levels of the amino acid homocysteine suggests that increasing the amount of folates we get from diet or adding a B vitamin supplement may offer added protection.

The bottom line? While vitamins and minerals (with the exception of calcium) have yet to be proven effective in alleviating or reversing the signs of menopause, they can be invaluable in maintaining health and vibrancy as we grow older. Older women, like older men, often do not eat as well as they should. We may live alone and hate to cook for one. Our fixed incomes may not stretch to cover a wide variety of healthful foods. We may not have the appetite we once enjoyed because we are not as active. Or we may simply forget to eat. All of these are reasons for choosing a good, basic, RDA-level vitamin and mineral supplement to keep us in nutritional balance.

BRAND NAME VITAMIN AND MINERAL PRODUCTS FOR WOMEN

For those of us who choose to take vitamin and mineral supplements, American drugstores present a dizzying variety of products. For safety's sake, it makes sense to stick close to the RDAs except, of course, when your doctor prescribes a specific product or combination to treat a particular condition.

MULTIVITAMIN AND MINERAL PRODUCTS

The choice includes widely promoted national brand-name products and those made and marketed by smaller, regional brands. As long as the ingredients and amounts are the same and the company reputable, the products provide similar benefits. As with generic versus brand name drugs, price and packaging are not necessarily an indication of value.

The most popular form of vitamin supplement is a tablet, "caplet," or capsule such as ONE-A-DAY, which provides multiple vitamins, or CENTRUM, which provides multiple vitamins and selected minerals in RDA amounts. Products labeled "women's supplement" generally add calcium and iron to the usual vitamins. "High potency" products such as STRESSTABS, THERAGRAN, VICON FORTE, or ZYMACAP may contain larger amounts of some nutrients. There appears to be no harm—and may be much benefit—from taking a basic RDA-level multivitamin or multivitamin/multimineral combination.

MENSTRUATION

For women of childbearing age, iron supplements provide insurance against iron-deficiency anemia due to the loss of blood and iron during menstrual bleeding. These tablets contain one of several iron compounds such as ferrous fumarate, ferrous gluconate, or ferrous sulfate. Because the compounds provide different amounts of *elemental iron,* the form of iron your body can absorb, the package label may list both the active ingredient and the amount of elemental iron. For example:

Ferrous gluconate 500 mg

Elemental iron 34 mg

This tells you that the iron compound in the product is 500 mg of *ferrous gluconate,* which supplies 34 mg of *elemental iron.* In multivitamin and mineral products, the word *iron* always stands for "elemental iron." Many iron supplements also contain vitamin C to improve your ability to absorb and use the iron.

Oral contraceptives appear to increase the need for B vitamins, so if you are using birth control pills, your doctor may suggest a multi-B supplement. Some B-vitamin supplements also contain vitamin C.

PREGNANCY

Vitamin and mineral supplements for a pregnant woman are similar to basic multivitamin, multimineral supplements, with slightly higher amounts of many nutrients to supply the needs of the growing fetus. These products may also be useful while you are nursing.

MENOPAUSE

Calcium supplements are an important nutritional tool for older women. The calcium compound most commonly found in supplements is calcium carbonate, which comes from limestone or crushed oyster shells. Other calcium compounds used in supplements are calcium citrate, calcium gluconate, and calcium lactate. As with iron, the different calcium compounds supply different amounts of elemental calcium, the form of calcium our bodies absorb. Therefore, the product label usually shows the active calcium compound (for example, calcium carbonate) along with the amount of elemental calcium it supplies. Anytime the word *calcium* appears alone, it means elemental calcium.

One note of caution: some antacids, such as TUMS, are made of calcium carbonate and may be used as calcium supplements. However, other antacids may contain magnesium or aluminum compounds. *Magnesium and aluminum antacids are not vitamin or mineral supplements. They are designed solely as antacids to relieve digestive upset. Never assume that an antacid can be used as a calcium supplement. Always check the label first.*

Pages 147–151 contain charts comparing selected supplements of multinutrients, iron, and B vitamins. The chart on pages 152–153 compares selected vitamins and minerals for pregnant women, and the chart on pages 154–155 compares calcium sources.

COMPARING THE PRODUCTS: SELECTED MULTINUTRIENT SUPPLEMENTS*

	One-A-Day essential vitamins (Miles)	One-A-Day maximum multivitamin multimineral (Miles)	One-A-Day women's (Miles)
Nutrient	*Amount*		
Vitamin A	5,000 IU	5,000 IU	5,000 IU
Vitamin D	400 IU	400 IU	400 IU
Vitamin E	30 IU	30 IU	30 IU
Vitamin C	60 mg	60 mg	60 mg
Thiamin (vitamin B1)	1.5 mg	1.5 mg	1.5 mg
Riboflavin (vitamin B2)	1.7 mg	1.7 mg	1.7 mg
Niacin	20 mg	20 mg	20 mg
Vitamin B6	2 mg	2 mg	2 mg
Folate	0.4 mg	0.4 mg	0.4 mg
Vitamin B12	6 mcg	6 mcg	6 mcg
Pantothenic Acid	10 mg	10 mg	10 mg
Calcium	—	130 mg	450 mg
Iron	—	18 mg	27 mg
Phosphorus	—	100 mg	—
Iodine	—	150 mcg	—
Magnesium	—	100 mg	—
Copper	—	2 mg	—
Zinc	—	15 mg	15 mg
Chromium	—	10 mcg	—

	One-A-Day essential vitamins (Miles)	One-A-Day maximum multivitamin multimineral (Miles)	One-A-Day women's (Miles)
Nutrient	*Amount*		
Selenium	—	10 mcg	—
Molybdenum	—	10 mcg	—
Manganese	—	2.5 mg	—
Potassium	—	37.5 mg	—
Chloride	—	34 mg	—

* For purposes of comparison, this chart shows three products from the same company. Similar combinations are available from other companies.

Sources: Products on sale in New York City, summer 1995. *Physicians' Desk Reference for Nonprescription Drugs,* 16th ed. (Montvale, NJ: Medical Economics Data, 1995).

COMPARING THE PRODUCTS: SELECTED IRON SUPPLEMENTS

Product (Supplier)	Elemental Iron per Dose (Iron Compound)	Other Nutrients
FEOSOL CAPSULES (SmithKline Beecham)	50 mg (ferrous sulfate)	
FEOSOL ELIXIR (SmithKline Beecham)	44 mg (ferrous sulfate)	
FEOSOL TABLETS (SmithKline Beecham)	65 mg (ferrous sulfate)	
FERANCEE CHEWABLE TABLETS (Johnson & Johnson-Merck)	134 mg (ferrous sulfate)	vitamin C, 300 mg
FERANCEE-HP (Johnson & Johnson-Merck)	110 mg (ferrous fumarate)	vitamin C, 600 mg
FERGON TABLETS (Miles)	36 mg (ferrous gluconate)	
FERO-FOLIC 500 FILMTAB (Abbott)	105 mg (ferrous sulfate)	vitamin C, 500 mg folic acid, 800 mcg
FERO-GRAD 500 FILMTAB (Abbott)	105 mg (ferrous sulfate)	vitamin C, 500 mg
FERO-GRADUMET FILMTAB (Abbott)	105 mg (ferrous sulfate)	vitamin C, 500 mg
FERRO SEQUELS (Lederle)	50 mg (ferrous fumarate)	
IBERET FOLIC 500 LIQUID (Abbott)	26.25 mg (ferrous sulfate)	vitamin C, 600 mg niacinamide, 30 mg thiamin, 6 mg riboflavin, 6 mg folic acid, 600 mcg vitamin B12, 25 mcg pantothenic acid (calcium pantothenate), 10 mg

Product (Supplier)	Elemental Iron per Dose (Iron Compound)	Other Nutrients
NU-IRON 150 CAPSULES (Mayrand)	150 mg (polysaccharide iron complex)	
NU-IRON ELIXIR (Mayrand)	100 mg (polysaccharide iron complex)	
NU-IRON PLUS ELIXIR (Mayrand)	100 mg (polysaccharide iron complex)	folic acid, 1 mg vitamin B12, 25 mcg
SLOW FE (Ciba)	50 mg (ferrous sulfate)	
SLOW FE WITH FOLIC ACID (Ciba)	50 mg (ferrous sulfate)	folic acid, 400 mcg
STUARTINIC CAPSULES (Johnson & Johnson-Merck)	100 mg (ferrous fumarate)	vitamin C, 500 mg thiamin, 4.9 mg riboflavin, 6 mg niacin, 20 mg vitamin B6, 0.8 mg vitamin 12, 25 mcg pantothenic acid 9.2 mg
VITRON C (Ciba)	66 mg (ferrous fumarate)	vitamin C, 125 mg

Sources: Physicians' Desk Reference, 48th ed. (Montvale, NJ: Medical Economics Data, 1994). Physicians' Desk Reference for Nonprescription Drugs, 16th ed. (Montvale, NJ: Medical Economics Data, 1995). Products on sale in New York City, summer 1995.

COMPARING THE PRODUCTS:
SELECTED B VITAMIN SUPPLEMENTS

Product (Supplier)	Vit B1 (mg)	Vit B2 (mg)	Niacin (mg)	Folate (mg)	Vit B6 (mg)	Vit B12 (mcg)	Panto-thenic acid (mg)	Vit C (mg)
APATATE LIQUID/TABLETS (Kenwood)	15	—	—	—	0.5	25	—	—
BEROCCA (Roche)	15	15	100	0.5	18	5	18	500
CEFOL* (Abbott)	15	10	100	0.5	5	6	20	750
IBERET-500[†] (Abbott)	1.5	1.5	7.5	—	1.25	6.25	2.5	125
MEGA-B** (Arco)	100	100	100	100	100	100	100	—

* also contains 30 IU vitamin E

† also contains 26.25 mg ferrous sulfate (elemental iron)

** also contains 100 mg biotin; 100 mg PABA

Sources: *Physicians' Desk Reference,* 48th ed. (Montvale, NJ: Medical Economics Data, 1994). *Physicians' Desk Reference for Nonprescription Drugs,* 16th ed. (Montvale, NJ: Medical Economics Data, 1995). Products on sale in New York City, summer 1995.

COMPARING THE PRODUCTS: SELECTED VITAMINS/MINERALS FOR PREGNANT WOMEN

Product (Supplier)	Vit A IU*	Vit D IU*	Vit E IU*	Vit C mg	Folic acid mg	B1 mg	B2 mg	Nia-cin mg	B6 mg	B12 mcg
MATERNA† (Lederle)	5,000	400	30	100	1.0	3.0	3.4	20	10	12
NATALINS (Mead Johnson)	4,000	400	15	70	0.5	1.5	1.6	17	2.6	2.5
NATALINS RX** (Mead Johnson)	4,000	400	15	80	1.0	1.5	1.6	17	4.0	2.5
NESTABS FA (Fielding)	5,000	400	30	120	1.0	3.0	3.0	20	3	8
NIFEREX-PN (Central Pharmaceuticals)	4,000	400	—	50	1.0	3.0	3.0	10	2	3
PRAMILET FA†† (Ross)	4,000	400	—	60	1.0	3.0	2.0	10	3	3
STUARTNATAL 1+1 (Wyeth-Ayerst)	4,000	400	11	120	1.0	1.5	3	20	10	12
STUART PRENATAL (Wyeth-Ayerst)	4,000	400	11	100	0.8	1.5	1.7	18	2.6	4.0
ZENATE (Solvay)	5,000	400	30	80	1.0	3.0	3	20	10	12

(Table continues on facing page)

Product (Supplier)	Calcium (mg)	Iodine (mcg)	Iron (mg)	Magnesium (mg)	Copper (mg)	Zinc (mg)
MATERNA† (Lederle)	250	150	60	25	2	25
NATALINS (Mead Johnson)	200	—	30	100	1.5	15
NATALINS RX** (Mead Johnson)	200	—	60	100	3	25
NESTABS FA (Fielding)	500	150	100	—	—	15
NIFEREX-PN (Central Pharmaceuticals)	125	—	60	—	—	18
PRAMILET FA†† (Ross)	250	100	40	10	0.15	0.085
STUARTNATAL 1+1 (Wyeth-Ayerst)	200	—	65	—	2	25
STUART PRENATAL (Wyeth-Ayerst)	200	—	60	—	—	25
ZENATE (Solvay)	300	175	65	100	—	20

* Product labels use IU for vitamins A, D, and E.

† Also contains 30 mcg biotin, 10 mg pantothenic acid, 25 mcg chromium, 25 mcg molybdenum, 5 mg manganese

** Also contains 30 mcg biotin, 7 mg pantothenic acid

†† Also contains 1 mg calcium pantothenate (pantothenic acid)

Sources: Physicians' Desk Reference, 48th ed. (Montvale, NJ: Medical Economics Data, 1994). Physicians' Desk Reference for Nonprescription Drugs, 16th ed. (Montvale, NJ: Medical Economics Data, 1995). Products on sale in New York City, summer 1995.

COMPARING THE PRODUCTS:
SELECTED CALCIUM SOURCES*

Product (Supplier)	Product Type	Amount of Elemental Calcium Per Tablet	Form of Calcium, Other Nutrients
ALKA-MINTS (Miles)	antacid chewable	340 mg	calcium carbonate
CALTRATE 600 (Lederle)	supplement	600 mg	calcium carbonate
CALTRATE 600+D (Lederle)	supplement	600 mg	calcium carbonate vitamin D, 200 IU
CALTRATE PLUS (Lederle)	supplement	600 mg	calcium carbonate vitamin D, 400 IU magnesium, 40 mg copper, 1 mg manganese, 1.6 mg zinc, 7.5 mg
CENTRUM SINGLES CALCIUM (Lederle)	supplement	500 mg	calcium carbonate
CHOOZ (Schering Plough)	antacid gum	200 mg	calcium carbonate
DICAL-D (Abbott)	supplement tablets	350 mg	dibasic calcium phosphate vitamin D, 399 IU phosphorus, 270 mg
DICAL-D (Abbott)	supplement wafers	464 mg	dibasic calcium phosphate vitamin D, 400 IU phosphorus, 360 mg
OSCAL (SmithKline Beecham)	supplement	500 mg	calcium carbonate
OSCAL CHEWABLE (SmithKline Beecham)	supplement	500 mg	calcium carbonate

Product (Supplier)	Product Type	Amount of Elemental Calcium Per Tablet	Form of Calcium, Other Nutrients
OSCAL 500+ VITAMIN D (SmithKline Beecham)	supplement	500 mg	calcium carbonate vitamin D, 125 mg
ROLAIDS ORIGINAL (Warner Lambert)	antacid	165 mg	calcium carbonate
ROLAIDS CALCIUM RICH/SODIUM FREE (Warner Lambert)	antacid	220 mg	calcium carbonate
TUMS ASSORTED FLAVORS (SmithKline Beecham)	antacid	200 mg	calcium carbonate
TUMS E-X (SmithKline Beecham)	antacid	300 mg	calcium carbonate
TUMS ULTRA (SmithKline Beecham)	antacid	400 mg	calcium carbonate
TUMS 500 CALCIUM SUPPLEMENT (SmithKline Beecham)	supplement	500 mg	calcium carbonate

* Calcium values apply to the products named. Other products with the same brand name may not provide calcium or may not provide the amount specified here.

Sources: Physicians' Desk Reference, 48th ed. (Montvale, NJ: Medical Economics Data, 1994). *Physician's Desk Reference for Nonprescription Drugs*, 16th ed. (Montvale, NJ: Medical Economics Data, 1995). "Calcium," *Consumer Reports*, August 1995. Products on sale in New York City, summer 1995.

SOURCES

Altman, Lawrence, "Study finds a vitamin reduces birth defects," *New York Times,* July 19, 1991.

"Anemia may be cause of some women's cold sensitivity," *Science News,* June 13, 1988.

Boston Women's Health Book Collective, *The New Our Bodies, Ourselves* (New York: Touchstone, 1992).

Briggs, George M., and Doris Howes Callaway, *Nutrition and Physical Fitness,* 11th ed. (New York: Holt, Rinehart and Winston, 1984).

Brody, Jane, "Sorting out the benefits of taking extra vitamin E," *New York Times,* July 20, 1995.

"Calcium: Make no bones about it," Food Information Council Foundation, September/October 1994.

Farb, Peter, and George Armelagos, *Consuming Passions: The Anthropology of Eating* (New York: Houghton Mifflin, 1980).

"Food and drugs," *Mayo Clinic Health Letter,* April 1991.

"Health Gazette/Medical News (smoking and vitamin C)," *U.S. Pharmacist,* February 1994.

Ivey, Marianne, and Gary Elmer, "Nutritional supplements, mineral, and vitamin products," *Handbook of Nonprescription Drugs*, 9th ed. (Washington, DC: American Pharmaceutical Association, 1990).

Kolata, Gina, "Advice unheeded on averting birth defects," *New York Times*, March 4, 1995.

Long, James W., and James J. Rybacki, *The Essential Guide to Prescription Drugs 1995* (New York: HarperCollins, 1995).

The Merck Manual, 16th ed. (Rahway, NJ: Merck Research Laboratories, 1992).

Morgan, Brian L. G., *The Food and Drug Interaction Guide* (New York: Simon and Schuster, 1986).

National Research Council, *Recommended Dietary Allowances,* 10th ed. (Washington, DC: National Academy Press, 1989).

"Optimal calcium intake," *NIH Consensus Statement* V.12, N.4 (Bethesda, MD: National Institutes of Health, June 6–8, 1994).

Physicians' Desk Reference, 48th ed. (Montvale, NJ: Medical Economics Data, 1994).

Physicians' Desk Reference for Nonprescription Drugs, 16th ed. (Montvale, NJ: Medical Economics Data, 1995).

Quarterly Report of Selected Research Projects, Agricultural Research Service, U.S. Department of Agriculture: vitamin B6, calcium/menstruation, April–June 1991; vitamin C and t3 levels, January–March 1992; homocysteine and brain cells, January–March 1993; vitamin E from diet alone, April–June 1993; vegetarian riboflavin requirements, April–June 1994; vitamin C and cholesterol, January–March 1995.

Rinzler, Carol Ann, "Food fights," *MOXIE,* July 1990.

"Smoking depletes vitamin C from mom, fetus," *Science News,* May 20, 1995.

"Study ties extra zinc to larger, healthier babies," *New York Times,* August 9, 1995.

U.S. Department of Agriculture/Human Nutrition Information Service, "Good sources of nutrients," pamphlet, Washington, DC: January 1990.

Wilson, Jean D., et al., eds., *Harrison's Principles of Internal Medicine, 12th ed. (New York: McGraw Hill, 1991).*

CHAPTER 5

DIET AND WEIGHT-CONTROL PRODUCTS

PRESCRIPTION DRUGS FOR WEIGHT CONTROL

Like many successful products, prescription appetite suppressants (also known as anorectics) began life as something else entirely. Early in the 1930s, researchers discovered that amphetamines were effective central nervous system stimulants with a promising ability to treat depression or narcolepsy, the disorder that causes people to fall asleep involuntarily many times a day. In was not until the amphetamines had been in use for several years that someone cataloguing their side effects—wakefulness, nervousness, shakiness—found a marketable one on the list: loss of appetite.

Soon, controlled studies showed that people taking amphetamines lost weight more quickly than dieters relying on "will power" alone, and the amphetamines were off and running.

At the height of their popularity in the 1950s, amphetamine sulfate (BENZEDRINE) and dextroamphetamine (DEXEDRINE) were available virtually for the asking from family practitioners. With minimal controls and an increasing number of pills in circulation, many people discovered that taking amphetamines not only helped them control their weight but also made them feel brighter and think faster, at least temporarily. Students cramming for exams, athletes racing for a new record, truck drivers plowing through a 24-hour day on the road, housewives trapped in the impossible dream of a perfect home—all learned to reach for the diet pill that promised instant energy and instant smarts.

Did the pills make a person irritable? agitated? disoriented? No matter. In the drug revolution of the 1960s, the side effects that made amphetamines unacceptable to many dieters came to be regarded as tolerable, even welcome, for those seeking a high. By the middle of the decade, methamphetamine, commonly known as "speed," ranked among the most popular of the "recreational drugs."

NEW DRUG REGULATIONS

The resulting abuse forced a serious reexamination of the laws regarding the availability of a number of drugs, including amphetamines. In 1970, the federal government created a new set of guidelines, the Controlled Substances Act of 1970. It classifies drugs according to how likely they are to create physical or psychological dependence. Obviously, the higher the potential for dependence, the higher the potential for abuse. Not surprisingly, the amphetamines and some amphetamine-like drugs ranked high in both categories.

Once the new law was in place, prescribing amphetamines became more difficult, and their use declined. But that did not cure the problem. The reduced availability of amphetamines led to the creation of a new generation of appetite suppressants, chemical cousins of amphetamines such as diethylpropion (TENUATE), mazindol (SANOREX), and phendimetrazine (BONTRIL, PLEGINE, PRELU-2). Many people assumed that these drugs would be less troublesome than the amphetamines, but in fact the only difference was that they were slightly less likely to cause physical or psychological dependence. The third generation of appetite suppressants, fenfluramine (PONDIMIN) and phentermine (ADIPEX, IONAMIN), do not seem—as of this writing—to cause dependence, *but* using PONDIMIN or a related drug, REDUX (desfenfluramine), increases the risk of a life-threatening lung disorder, primary pulmonary hypertension.

Nonetheless, all prescription appetite suppressants share a number of unpleasant side effects (see pages 161–165 for a list):

- All may create a tolerance, meaning that you need increasing amounts to produce the same effect.

- All may cause gastric upset including diarrhea, constipation, and vomiting.

- All may affect libido, reducing or increasing your desire for sex.

- Most are central nervous system stimulants that can make you jumpy or irritable and keep you up at night. (The exception is fenfluramine, which depresses rather than stimulates the central nervous system.)

- When given in very large doses to laboratory animals, most have been shown to cause birth defects or fetal death in one or more species.

- Most are known to be excreted in breast milk.

FUTURE SKINNY

In the spring of 1995, the continuing search for the perfect appetite suppressant and weight-control medication produced two interesting new possibilities, a drug that blocks the brain's natural production of opiates (heroinlike chemicals) and a hormone that appears to slim down fat mice.

At the University of Michigan School of Public Health in Ann Arbor, a team of nutritionists enlisted 41 women as volunteers in a study designed to see if a drug blocking normal opiate production controls appetite. There were 16 obese women and 25 women of normal weight; 10 from each group were diagnosed with either bulimia or a binge-eating disorder. The women were randomly chosen to get a 2.5-hour infusion of either naloxone (a drug that blocks the action of opiates produced naturally in the brain), salt water, or butorphanol (a drug that both blocks and strengthens the action of naturally produced opiates). Before the infusions began and 1 hour into the test, the women were asked to rate their preferences for sweet and fatty foods. While naloxone did not affect taste perceptions, it did reduce the amount of fats and sweets consumed by women diagnosed as binge eaters. In other words, the drug lowered the pleasurable reinforcement that natural brain chemicals provided binge eaters and showed that breaking the addictive cycle may be useful in treating people with eating disorders.

The second big story of spring 1995 was leptin, a hormone produced by a mouse gene. In 1950, a spontaneous mutation in a mouse gene produced a colony of extremely overweight mice at the Jackson Laboratory in Bar Harbor, Maine. It has taken nearly half a century, but scientists at the Howard Hughes Medical Institute at Rockefeller University in New York have now shown that a hormone, leptin, produced by the *unmutated* version of this gene slims down mice whose obesity comes from either their genes or a high-fat diet. The researchers have also shown that leptin is made by a human gene for obesity, so the question now on the table is whether, at long last, there will be a magic pill for fat control.

THE CONTROLLED SUBSTANCES ACT OF 1970: DRUG CLASSIFICATIONS

Category	Examples	Description
I	heroin, marijuana	These have a high potential for abuse and physical and psychological dependence. They are used only for research and cannot legally be prescribed as medicines.
II	morphine, codeine (alone), amphetamines	These also have a high potential for abuse and may lead to severe physical or psychological dependence. However, they are legal for use as medicines. A prescription in ink (or typewritten) and signed by a physician is required. Telephone orders, allowed only in emergency, must be confirmed in writing within 72 hours. No refills are permitted; a second use requires a new written prescription.
III	codeine, hydrocodone, or paregoric in combination with a non-narcotic drug such as acetaminophen	These have a potential for abuse, but less than category II drugs. Using them may lead to low-to-moderate dependence or high psychological dependence. The prescription may be written or called in to the pharmacist who then puts it in written form. Up to 5 refills are allowed within a 6-month period. After that, you need a new written prescription.
IV	propoxyphene (DARVON), benzodiazapines (LIBRIUM, VALIUM)	These have a lower potential for abuse than category III drugs, but using them may lead to physical or psychological dependence. The prescription may be written or telephoned to the pharmacist. Up to 5 refills are allowed within a 6-month period. After that, you need a new written prescription.
V	diphenoxylate (LOMOTIL)	These carry a low risk of abuse; they may be regulated by state and local governments and can be sold without a prescription, over the counter.

Sources: James W. Long and James J. Rybacki, *The Essential Guide to Prescription Drugs 1995* (New York: HarperCollins, 1995). *Physicians' Desk Reference,* 48th ed. (Montvale, NJ: Medical Economics Data, 1994).

COMPARING THE PRODUCTS:
PRESCRIPTION APPETITE SUPPRESSANTS
AMPHETAMINES AND AMPHETAMINE-LIKE DRUGS

Product (Supplier)	Active Ingredient	Category	Possible Side Effects	Reproductive Effects
ADIPEX-P (Gate)	Phentermine	IV	High blood pressure, fast or irregular heartbeat, psychotic episodes, dizziness, elation, insomnia, shakiness, restlessness, headache, stomach upset (diarrhea or constipation), dry mouth, odd or unpleasant taste in mouth, hives, increase or decrease in sexual desire.	Safe use in pregnancy has not been established.
BONTRIL PDM (Carnrick)	Phen-dimetrazine; timed-release	III	See ADIPEX-P.	Safe use in pregnancy has not been established.
DESOXYN (Abbott)	metham-phetamine; timed-release	II	See ADIPEX-P.	When given in large doses, causes birth defects and fetal death in laboratory animals; no adequate studies in humans available. However, babies born to women who take this drug while pregnant are at increased risk of prematurity and low birthweight and may show withdrawal symptoms after birth. Amphetamines are excreted in a nursing mother's milk.

Product (Supplier)	Active Ingredient	Category	Possible Side Effects	Reproductive Effects
DEXE-DRINE (Smith-Kline Beecham)	Dextro-amphetamine; timed-release	II	See ADIPEX-P.	Caused birth defects and fetal death when given to laboratory mice in doses 41 times the maximum human dose; these effects were not seen in rats or rabbits given, respectively, 12.5 and 7 times the maximum human dose. Similar studies in human beings are not available, but babies born to women who take this drug while pregnant are more likely to be born premature or low birthweight.
DIDREX (Upjohn)	Benzphet-amine	III	See ADIPEX-P. Note: The 25 mg tablet contains FD&C Yellow #5 (tartrazine), which may cause allergic reactions in susceptible individuals, particularly those sensitive to aspirin.	May be harmful to the fetus. Excreted in breast milk.
FASTIN (Smith-Kline Beecham)	Phentermine	IV	See ADIPEX-P.	Safe use in pregnancy has not been established.
IONAMIN (Fisons)	Phentermine	IV	See ADIPEX-P.	Safe use in pregnancy has not been established.

Product (Supplier)	Active Ingredient	Category	Possible Side Effects	Reproductive Effects
OBETROL (Rexar)	Dextro-amphetamine and amphetamine	II	See ADIPEX-P. Note: The 20 mg tablet contains FD&C Yellow #6 (sunset yellow FCF), which may cause allergic reactions, including bronchial asthma, in susceptible people, particularly those sensitive to aspirin.	See DEXEDRINE.
PLEGINE (Wyeth-Ayerst)	Phendi-metrazine	III	See ADIPEX-P.	Safe use in pregnancy has not been established.
PONDA-MIN (Robins)	Fenfluramine	IV	The most common side effects are drowsiness, diarrhea, and dry mouth. Other possible side effects: Dizziness, confusion, loss of coordination, nervousness, insomnia, weakness, fatigue, changes in libido, agitation, constipation, nausea, abdominal pain, sweating, chills, blurred vision, painful or frequent urination, changes in blood pressure, heart palpitations, rashes, hives, burning sensation on skin, fever, irritated eyes, chest pain, unpleasant taste in mouth.	Caused reduced rates of conception and possible damage to the fetus in rats at doses 20 times the customary human dose. However, these effects did not occur in rats, rabbits, mice, and monkeys at doses up to, respectively, 5, 20, 1, and 5 times the dose prescribed for humans. It is not known whether this drug is excreted in breast milk.

Product (Supplier)	Active Ingredient	Category	Possible Side Effects	Reproductive Effects
PRELU-2 (Boehringer Ingelheim)	Phendi-metrazine; timed-release	III	See ADIPEX-P. Note: Contains FD&C Yellow #6, (sunset yellow FCF), which may cause allergic reactions, including bronchial asthma, in susceptible people, particularly those sensitive to aspirin.	Safe use in pregnancy has not been established.
SANOREX (Sandoz)	Mazindol	IV	See ADIPEX-P. Note: Laboratory dogs given high doses for long periods of time developed corneal opacity (cataracts), which disappeared when the drug was discontinued; no such effect has been observed in human beings.	Relatively high doses given to laboratory rats and rabbits caused an increase in neonatal deaths and a possible increased incidence in fetal birth defects (rib abnormalities). The extent to which this drug is excreted in human breast milk is unknown.
TENUATE and TENUATE DOSPAN (Marion Merrell Dow)	Diethyl-propion; immediate release (TENUATE); controlled release (TENUATE DOSPAN)	IV	See ADIPEX-P. Other side effects: Increase in epileptic seizures, bone marrow depression, blood abnormalities, painful or excessive urination, shortness of breath, hair loss, muscle pain, increased sweating.	Reproductive studies with laboratory rats given 9 times the customary human dose have shown no evidence of reduced fertility or harm to the fetus. However, there are no adequate studies in human beings. This drug is excreted in human breast milk.

Sources: James W. Long, and James J. Rybacki, *The Essential Guide to Prescription Drugs 1995* (New York: HarperCollins, 1995). *Physicians' Desk Reference*, 48th ed. (Montvale, NJ: Medical Economics Data, 1994).

NONPRESCRIPTION APPETITE SUPPRESSANTS

In 1970, when the federal government began to tighten the regulations governing prescription appetite suppressants, the most popular nonprescription diet product was AYDS, a candy meant to dull the appetite by satisfying the natural craving for sweets. Take one AYDS before meals, the promotion went, and you'll be less hungry, eat less, and lose weight. It was a nice idea, but not very effective, and soon the over-the-counter diet market switched from a candy to a drug, phenylpropanolamine.

PHENYLPROPANOLAMINE DIET PILLS

Phenylpropanolamine is the active ingredient in many appetite suppressants. It is also used as a decongestant in such popular allergy and cold pills as ALLEREST 12 HOUR, COMTREX MULTI-SYMPTOM, CONTAC MAXIMUM STRENGTH CONTINUOUS ACTION, and TAVIST-D 12 HOUR.

Despite its popularity, the evidence as to phenylpropanolamine's effectiveness in suppressing appetite seems mixed. Some studies say it works well, others that it produces only a small weight loss. In 1982, an FDA advisory review panel on miscellaneous internal drug products rated it safe and effective for short-term dieting, setting the dosages at 37.5 mg in "immediate release" products and 75 mg in "timed release" products that give day-long control.

NONDRUG DIET PILLS

Some diet pills are actually diuretics or laxatives. Their active ingredients are diuretic herbs such as dandelion root, laxatives such as psyllium, or irritants such as cayenne pepper along with vitamins and minerals.

Strictly speaking, diuretics are of no real value when you are trying to lose weight. They do produce a temporary loss of water so that you weigh less, but you will regain that quickly. These products do not suppress appetite or "burn fat."

SIDE EFFECTS AND INTERACTIONS

Although diet pills are available without prescription, they are serious medicine and should not be used without your doctor's advice, particularly if you have a chronic medical condition other than obesity.

PHENYLPROPANOLAMINE PRODUCTS   Controlled clinical studies have shown that phenylpropanolamine appears safe in healthy people, but it is not without side effects. Phenylpropanolamine is not an amphetamine, but it has some similar effects. For example, it constricts blood vessels, which is why it is useful in shrinking swollen nasal tissues but hazardous for someone with high blood pressure or heart disease. It is a weak central nervous system stimulant that can cause headache, nausea, restlessness, agitation, shakiness, and insomnia even in normal doses. There have been some reports of psychotic episodes in people taking phenylpropanolamine, but overall the incidence of side effects is far less than with any of the prescription anorectics. Like the amphetamines and their relatives, phenylpropanolamine is excreted in human breast milk. There have been reports of high blood pressure linked to use of phenylpropanolamine, but this appears to be less likely with timed-release products. Amphetamine-like reactions including seizures, respiratory problems, agitation, and hallucination have also been observed from either phenylpropanolamine alone or in combination with caffeine or ephedrine. Both combinations, formerly widely available, were declared "unapproved new drug products" and removed from the market in 1982.

Phenylpropanolamine interacts with monoamine oxidase inhibitors while you are taking it and for some time after. It elevates blood sugar levels, makes blood vessels contract, and stimulates heart function, making it potentially hazardous for people with diabetes, high blood pressure, or heart disease. Its ability to constrict blood vessels (the basis for its use in decongestants) may make it dangerous for people with high blood pressure, heart disease, or a thyroid disorder.

DIURETICS AND LAXATIVES   If used to excess or without sufficient liquids, diuretics are dehydrating. The same is true of laxatives, which can also upset the stomach. Irritating ingredients such as cayenne pepper may increase urination, but they can also produce an uncomfortable, sometimes burning sensation.

COMPARING THE PRODUCTS: OTC DIET PILLS

Product (Supplier)	Appetite Suppressant	Other Ingredients
ACUTRIM (Ciba)	phenylpropanolamine 75 mg, timed-release	cellulose acetate, FD&C Yellow #10, FD&C Blue #1, FD&C Yellow #6, hydroxypropyl methycellulose, povidone, propylene glycol, stearic acid, titanium dioxide
ACUTRIM LATE DAY STRENGTH (Ciba)	phenylpropanolamine 75 mg, timed-release	cellulose acetate, FD&C Yellow #6, hydroxypropyl methycellulose, isopropyl alcohol, propylene glycol, riboflavin, stearic acid, titanium dioxide
ACUTRIM 16-HOUR STEADY CONTROL (Ciba)	phenylpropanolamine 75 mg, timed-release	cellulose acetate, hydroxypropyl methylcellulose, stearic acid
ADVANCED FORMULA GRAPE-FRUIT DIET (Fiske)	phenylpropanolamine 75 mg	natural grapefruit extract (no other ingredient listed)
DEXATRIM EXTENDED DURATION (Thompson Medical)	phenylpropanolamine 75 mg, timed-release	calcium sulfate, carnauba wax, FD&C Yellow #10 aluminum lake, ethylcellulose, FD&C Yellow #6, hydroxypropyl methylcellulose, iron oxide, magnesium stearate, stearic acid, titanium dioxide, triacetin
DEXATRIM MAXIMUM STRENGTH WITH VITAMIN C (Thompson Medical)	phenylpropanolamine 75 mg, timed-release	vitamin C (180 mg), carnauba wax, croscormellose sodium, ethylcellulose, FD&C Red #40 aluminum lake, hydroxypropyl methylcellulose, magnesium stearate, microcrystalline cellulose, polyethylene glycol, polysorbate 80, povidone, silicon dioxide, stearic acid, titanium dioxide

Product (Supplier)	Appetite Suppressant	Other Ingredients
DEXATRIM PLUS VITAMINS (Thompson Medical)	phenylpropanolamine 75 mg, timed-release	vitamin C (180 mg), croscormellose sodium, ethylcellulose, FD&C Red #40 aluminum lake, FD&C Yellow #6 aluminum lake, hydroxypropyl methyl-cellulose, magnesium stearate, polyethylene glycol, polysorbate 80, stearic acid, titanium dioxide. May contain calcium sulfate dihydrate, carnauba wax, FD&C Blue #1 aluminum lake, lactose, microcrystalline cellulose, povidone, silicon dioxide (comes with multivitamin pill).
ULTRA LEAN (Great American Nutrition)	—	brindell berry extract, dandelion root, horsetail, juniper berries, cayenne, betaine, iodine, potassium, magnesium, vanadyl sulfate, chromium
WEIDER FAT BURNER (Weider Nutrition Group)	—	chromium (200 mg), choline bitartrate (400 mg), inositol (200 mg), 1-methionine (75 mg), psyllium seed husks (500 mg), cinnamon powder (300 mg), mustard seed powder (300 mg), uva ursi extract (50 mg), cayenne (15 mg)

Source: Products on sale in New York City, summer 1995.

FORMULA WEIGHT-LOSS DIET PRODUCTS

Deciding to go on a diet is easy. Figuring out what to eat once you do can be hard. That is why formula diet powders, liquids, and bars are so popular: they eliminate the guesswork.

Formula diet products are milk-based, low-fat, low-cholesterol convenience foods. Their protein comes from milk powder or soy protein. They are made palatable with the addition of (1) natural and artificial sweeteners such as sugar, fructose, and aspartame, (2) cholesterol-free vegetable oils to provide "richness," and (3) texturizers such as malto-dextrin, thickeners such as guar gum, and emulsifiers such as carrageenan to create a satisfying "mouthfeel." All formula diet products are enriched with nutrients so that one serving provides between 1/6 and 1/3 of the recommended dietary allowances (RDAs) of various vitamins and minerals based on a 2,000-calorie diet.

POWDERS

Protein-based powder supplements such as TIGER'S MILK were a staple in health food stores for years before the general public discovered premeasured meals. Unlike the earlier powders, whose flavors were often described as malty or faintly medicinal, the current crop comes in a variety such as chocolate, coffee, "French vanilla" banana, apple-cranberry-raspberry, and orange pineapple. For people who hate milk, there's an unflavored version to be mixed with fruit juice. The chief virtue of the powders may be that they give you the illusion of having some control over what you're eating because you get to mix the powder, shake it up, and "make" a meal.

LIQUIDS

Premeasured, flavored liquid meals first became popular in the early 1960s when METRACAL, the pioneer brand, was available in "soups" as well as "milk shakes." Current diet liquid products taste "fatter" than powders-plus-milk products. They have a texture some find satisfying; others, oily.

BARS

The forerunner of the current diet formula bar is the enriched chocolate "survival bar" packed into C-ration kits for GIs during World War II. Today's diet bar is less fatty but still very sweet. If your preference in a diet meal is tuna (hold the mayo) on plain rye with a tomato and lettuce salad, these may be too sweet for you.

HOW TO USE FORMULA DIET FOODS

No prepared formula diet product should replace an entire day's food supply, even when you are trying to lose weight quickly. Nor should you use these products without your doctor's advice. They may work well as substitutes for breakfast and/or lunch for short-term dieting as long as your third meal is well-balanced and nutritious. For long-term weight maintenance, however, it is far more sensible to learn how to handle calories and nutrients in real food. That way, at home or on the run, you can assemble a meal that provides the nutrients you need and satisfies your natural desire for taste and texture within healthful guidelines.

SUPPLEMENTS FOR WEIGHT GAIN OR EXTRA ENERGY

It is hard for those of us who have to diet to stay in shape to work up much sympathy for those who cannot gain weight, but the truth is that there are many women who would give their spiky hip bones for a layer of warm flesh over arm, thigh, and breast. The ingredients in ENSURE, NUTRAMENT, and SUSTACAL are similar to those in formula diet products, but these supplements provide more calories per serving to augment rather than reduce calorie consumption. The supplements are especially useful for older people or to round out a nutrient-deficient diet.

Powder mixes such as METAFORM, designed for people who work out, are similar to those for weight gain and weight loss but higher in calories and nutrients, providing 430 calories and more than 100% of the RDA for various vitamins and minerals when mixed with 16 ounces of nonfat milk or juice. They are also characteristically high in protein to build muscle tissue.

The charts on pages 172–180 compare the ingredients of a wide selection of formula foods.

COMPARING THE PRODUCTS:
SELECTED FORMULA FOODS

Product (Supplier)	Ingredients	Calories per Serving
POWDERS (WEIGHT-LOSS DIET)		
SWEET SUCCESS Dark Chocolate Fudge (Nestle)	Nonfat milk powder, sugar, cocoa, gum arabic, whey fudge powder concentrate, powdered diet formula cellulose, carrageenan, artificial colors (Red #40, Blue #1, Yellows #5 and 6), soy lecithin, aspartame, salt, natural and artificial flavors, malto-dextrin, cocoa powder.	90 (without milk); 180 (with 8 oz nonfat milk)

Nutritional profile per serving powder plus milk	
Calories from fat	10/15 with milk
Total fat	1.5 g
Saturated fat	1 g
Cholesterol	less than 5 mg
Sodium	210 mg
Potassium	—
Carbohydrates	19 g
Dietary fiber	6 g
Sugars	11 g
Protein	7 g

Vitamins and minerals per serving (% daily requirement based on a 2,000-calorie diet)

	Powder	Powder and milk
Vitamin A	25%	35%
Vitamin D	NA*	35%
Vitamin E	NA	35%
Vitamin C	35%	35%
Thiamin	NA	35%

Product (Supplier)	Ingredients		Calories per Serving
		Powder	Powder and milk	
	Riboflavin	NA	35%	
	Niacin	NA	35%	
	Vitamin B6	NA	35%	
	Folate	NA	35%	
	Vitamin B12	NA	35%	
	Biotin	NA	35%	
	Pantothenic acid	NA	35%	
	Calcium	20%	50%	
	Iron	35%	35%	
	Zinc	NA	35%	
	Phosphorus	NA	35%	
	Iodine	NA	35%	
	Magnesium	NA	35%	
	Copper	NA	35%	
	*NA = not available			
ULTRA SLIM FAST Lowfat Chocolate Malt Diet Formula (Slim Fast)	Sucrose, whey powder soy protein isolate, cocoa, powdered cellulose, fructose, corn bran, calcium caseinate, nonfat dry milk, guar gum, malt extract, carrageenan, natural and artificial flavors, soy lecithin, soy fiber, malto-dextrin, dextrose, aspartame.		110 (without milk); 200 (with 8 oz nonfat milk)
	Nutritional profile per serving powder plus milk		
	Calories from fat	10	
	Total fat	1 g	
	Saturated fat	0.5 mg	
	Cholesterol	less than 5 mg	
	Sodium	100 mg	
	Potassium	350 mg	

Product (Supplier)	Ingredients			Calories per Serving
	Carbohydrates	24 g		
	Dietary fiber	5 g		
	Sugars	17 g		
	Protein	5 g		
	Vitamins and minerals per serving (% daily requirement based on a 2,000-calorie diet)			
		Powder	*Powder and milk*	
	Vitamin A	50%	60%	
	Vitamin D	10%	35%	
	Vitamin E	50%	50%	
	Vitamin C	30%	35%	
	Thiamin	30%	35%	
	Riboflavin	15%	35%	
	Niacin	35%	35%	
	Vitamin B6	30%	35%	
	Folate	25%	30%	
	Vitamin B12	20%	35%	
	Biotin	35%	35%	
	Pantothenic acid	25%	35%	
	Calcium	15%	45%	
	Iron	35%	35%	
	Zinc	30%	35%	
	Phosphorus	10%	35%	
	Iodine	10%	35%	
	Magnesium	25%	30%	
	Copper	25%	25%	

Product (Supplier)	Ingredients	Calories per Serving
POWDER (HIGH PROTEIN, MUSCLE-BUILDING)		
METAFORM Chocolate (Great American Nutrition)	Milk protein isolate, caseinate, whey protein concentrate, egg albumin, cocoa, glucose polymers, cellulose gum, medium chain triglycerides, canola oil, natural and artificial flavors, dicalcium phosphate, guar gum, potassium chloride, dipotassium phosphate, magnesium oxide, potassium citrate, xanthan gum, choline bitartrate, sodium citrate, sodium chloride, aspartame, ascorbic acid, vitamin E acetate, inositol, molybdenum citrate, betaine hydrochloride, niacinamide, ferrous fumarate, vitamin A palmitate, selenium amino acid chelate, copper glutanate, PABA, manganese citrate, vitamin D3, pyridoxine hydrochloride, riboflavin, thiamin mononitrate, chromium picolenate, folic acid, biotin, potassium iodide, cyanocobalamin.	260 (without milk); 430 (with 8 oz nonfat milk)

Nutritional profile per serving powder plus milk

Calories from fat 20/25 with milk

Total fat	2 g
Saturated fat	1 g
Cholesterol	0 mg
Sodium	210 mg
Potassium	1130 mg
Carbohydrates	25 g
Dietary fiber	3 g
Sugars	15 g
Protein	37 g

Product (Supplier)	Ingredients			Calories per Serving
	Vitamins and minerals per serving (% daily requirement based on a 2,000-calorie diet)			
		Powder	Powder and milk	
	Vitamin A	70%	90%	
	Vitamin D	70%	120%	
	Vitamin E	70%	70%	
	Vitamin C	70%	90%	
	Thiamin	70%	80%	
	Riboflavin	70%	90%	
	Niacin	100%	100%	
	Vitamin B6	70%	80%	
	Folate	70%	80%	
	Vitamin B12	70%	110%	
	Biotin	70%	70%	
	Pantothenic acid	70%	90%	
	Calcium	70%	140%	
	Iron	40%	40%	

LIQUID (WEIGHT-LOSS DIET)

Product (Supplier)	Ingredients		Calories per Serving
SWEET SUCCESS Dark Chocolate Fudge (Nestle)	Nonfat milk, water, sugar, cocoa, calcium caseinate, gum arabic, cellulose gel, corn oil, caramel color, carrageenan, disodium phosphate, monoglycerides, dextrose, artificial flavors, Red #3, Yellow #6, Blue #1.		200 (10-fluid-oz can)
	Nutritional profile per serving		
	Calories from fat	30	
	Total fat	3 g	
	Saturated fat	1 mg	
	Cholesterol less than	5 mg	
	Sodium	220 mg	

Product (Supplier)	Ingredients		Calories per Serving
	Carbohydrates	38 g	
	Dietary fiber	6 g	
	Sugars	30 g	
	Protein	12 g	
	Vitamins and minerals per serving (% daily requirement based on a 2,000-calorie diet)		
	Vitamin A	35%	
	Vitamin D	35%	
	Vitamin E	35%	
	Vitamin C	35%	
	Thiamin	35%	
	Riboflavin	35%	
	Niacin	35%	
	Vitamin B6	35%	
	Folate	35%	
	Vitamin B12	35%	
	Biotin	35%	
	Pantothenic acid	35%	
	Calcium	50%	
	Iron	35%	
	Zinc	35%	
	Phosphorus	35%	
	Iodine	35%	
	Magnesium	35%	
	Copper	35%	

Product (Supplier)	Ingredients	Calories per Serving
LIQUID (WEIGHT-BUILDING)		
NUTRAMENT Banana Flavor Food Supplement (Mead Johnson)	Skim milk, sugar, partially hydrogenated soybean oil, corn syrup solids, soy protein isolate, sodium caseinate, calcium caseinate, magnesium chloride, magnesium phosphate, artificial flavor, carrageenan, soy lecithin, sodium ascorbate, ferrous sulfate, zinc sulfate, vitamin E acetate, artificial color (annatto), vitamin A palmitate, vitamin B hydrochloride, thiamin hydrochloride, folic acid, biotin, riboflavin, vitamin D3, vitamin B12.	360 (12-fluid-oz can)

Nutritional profile per serving	
Calories from fat	90
Total fat	10 g
Saturated fat	1.5 mg
Cholesterol	10 mg
Sodium	250 mg
Potassium	500 mg
Total carbohydrates	52 g
Dietary fiber	1 g
Sugars	43 g
Protein	10 g

Vitamins and minerals per serving (% daily requirement based on a 2,000-calorie diet)	
Vitamin A	35%
Vitamin D	35%
Vitamin E	35%
Vitamin C	35%
Thiamin	35%
Riboflavin	35%
Niacin	35%
Vitamin B6	35%

Product (Supplier)	Ingredients	Calories per Serving
	Vitamins and minerals per serving (% daily requirement based on a 2,000-calorie diet)	
	Folate	35%	
	Vitamin B12	35%	
	Biotin	35%	
	Pantothenic acid	35%	
	Calcium	50%	
	Iron	35%	
	Zinc	35%	
	Phosphorus	35%	
	Iodine	35%	
	Magnesium	35%	
	Copper	35%	
BAR (WEIGHT-LOSS DIET)		
SLIM FAST Breakfast Bar Blueberry Fat Free (Slim Fast)	Enriched bleached and unbleached flour, corn syrup, sugar, high fructose corn syrup, blueberries, cellulose, flaked corn, dehydrated apple pieces, glycerine, citric acid, salt, modified corn starch, natural and artificial flavors, baking soda, whey powder, dried egg whites, pectin, soy lecithin, monocalcium phosphate, potassium sorbate, sodium citrate, artificial color (Red #40, Blue #1).	170 (bar); 230 (bar plus 6 oz skim milk)
	Nutritional profile per serving (bar alone)	
	Calories from fat	0 g	
	Total fat	0 g	
	Saturated fat	0 g	
	Cholesterol less than	0 mg	
	Sodium	170 mg	
	Potassium	150 mg	
	Carbohydrates	39 g	
	Dietary fiber	2 g	

Product (Supplier)	Ingredients			Calories per Serving
	Nutritional profile per serving (bar alone)			
	Sugars	23 g		
	Protein	1 g		
	Vitamins and minerals per serving (% daily requirement based on a 2,000-calorie diet)			
		Bar	Bar with milk	
	Vitamin A	10%	15%	
	Vitamin D	20%	40%	
	Vitamin E	25%	25%	
	Vitamin C	25%	25%	
	Thiamin	10%	10%	
	Riboflavin	10%	25%	
	Niacin	25%	25%	
	Vitamin B6	25%	25%	
	Folate	25%	25%	
	Vitamin B12	10%	20%	
	Biotin	25%	25%	
	Pantothenic acid	25%	35%	
	Calcium	4%	25%	
	Iron	0%	0%	
	Zinc	10%	10%	
	Phosphorus	0%	15%	
	Iodine	0%	15%	
	Magnesium	0%	4%	

Source: Products on sale in New York City, summer 1995, 1996.

HOW TO READ THE NEW FOOD LABELS

No matter how nutritious the formula is, no prepared diet powder, liquid, or bar will ever be as tasty and satisfying as real food. At the same time, maintaining a healthful weight may be as important as eating nutritious foods. And therein lies the rub: how do you control your diet while eating what you like?

For some people, formula diet products provide a good answer. But virtually all experts agree that the key to permanent weight control is learning how to handle food in a healthful way. One invaluable tool for doing this is the new label that appears on all foods and food products sold in the United States.

WHAT THE LABEL SHOWS

The Nutrition Labeling and Education Act of 1990 requires that as of May 1994, all food sold in the United States carry a detailed label that is a dieter's dream. The new label has four basic components: (1) a Nutrition Facts table, (2) information about the % Daily Value, (3) a list of ingredients, and (4) health and nutrition claims. Each is designed to make it easier for ordinary consumers to put together a nutritious, well-balanced diet.

NUTRITION FACTS   This is an easy-to-read chart describing the nutrient content of the food in the context of an "ideal" 2,000-calorie-a-day diet. The chart

- describes one serving in real-life terms such as 1/2 cup or 1 tablespoon, and lists the number of servings in the container.

- shows the number of calories in a serving, as well as the number of calories from fat.

- shows the amount of total fat, saturated fat, cholesterol, sodium, total carbohydrates, dietary fiber, sugars, and protein in one serving (in grams or milligrams) as well as the % Daily Value for these nutrients plus vitamins A and C, calcium, and iron.

% DAILY VALUE   This measurement, based on a 2,000-calorie-a-day diet, allows you to compare products at a glance by showing you how much of the nutrient each food serving contains. For example, a food serving with 30 mg cholesterol provides 10 percent of the amount of cholesterol considered acceptable for someone consuming 2,000 calories a day; a food serving with 10 mg cholesterol provides only 3 percent of the daily allowance.

As a general rule of thumb, the % Daily Value is useful even when your diet provides slightly more or slightly fewer calories than the average 2,000 a day. For example, a food with 5 percent or less of the % Daily Value for a nutrient is considered "low" in that nutrient whether you consume 1,400, 2,000, or 2,500 calories a day. On the other hand, a food with 20 percent or more of the % Daily Value for a particular nutrient is considered to be "high" in that nutrient on any of these three calorie allowances.

INGREDIENT LIST   This is a complete list of everything in the product in descending order by weight. Even foods with well-accepted recipes, such as catsup and mayonnaise, must now list their ingredients in the label. Some ingredients must also include their pedigrees; that is, the labels must say where the ingredients come from so that people who are allergic to various foods or prefer to avoid some foods on religious grounds will have all the information they need. For example, a "coffee whitener" that contains caseinate must be described as a "milk derivative" so that people who are sensitive to milk products will know the whitener is not milk-free. In addition, color additives are now listed by name (for example, FD&C Blue #1 rather than "artificial colors").

HEALTH AND NUTRITION CLAIMS   Health experts agree that what we eat affects our total health and that certain foods may raise or lower our risk of a number of serious conditions, such as heart disease, high blood pressure, diabetes, and cancer.

The 1990 labeling law allows foods that meet specific nutritional standards to put certain FDA-approved health and nutrition claims on the package. First, food processors may use descriptive words such as "light" or "high." Second, they may describe the effects of the nutritional content. For example, a product marked "high" in calcium may explain that adequate calcium intake is linked to a lower risk of osteoporosis. Similarly, a product that is "low" in cholesterol may say that low cholesterol intake may reduce the risk of heart disease.

USING THE NEW FOOD LABEL

Clearly, these changes are an important tool for people who wish to watch their calorie intake. The serving sizes reflect what people actually eat and are in line with current nutritional guidelines such as the advice to include several half-cup servings of fruits and vegetables in a daily menu. The % Daily Value tells you at a glance whether a specific food is high or low in important nutrients and links this information to a set of scientifically valid health claims. These labels are already on prepared "real food" diet products such as WEIGHT WATCHERS. But their best value lies in the fact that they allow you to make your own real-life diet with variety, taste, and eating pleasure. Who could ask for anything more? See the chart on page 187 for an explanation of label terms.

FDA-APPROVED HEALTH CLAIMS

Nutrient	Claim
Calcium	lower risk of osteoporosis
Fat	higher risk of cancer
Saturated fat	higher risk of heart disease
Cholesterol	higher risk of heart disease
Fiber (fruits, vegetables, grains)	reduced risk of certain forms of cancer reduced risk of heart disease
Fruits and vegetables	reduced risk of certain forms of cancer
Sodium	higher risk of high blood pressure

Source: Food and Drug Administration, Food Safety and Inspection Service, "An introduction to the new food label" (Washington DC: USDA/DHHS Publication No. [FDA] 94-2271, October 1993).

LABEL TERMS

This term	...applied to these nutrients	...means the food has
free	fat saturated fat cholesterol sugarless calories	less than 0.5 g per serving less than 0.5 g per serving less than 0.5 g per serving less than 0.5 g per serving fewer than 5 per serving
low	fat saturated fat sodium cholesterol calories	3 g or less per serving 1 g or less per serving 140 mg or less per serving 20 mg or less per serving 40 or fewer per serving
reduced	calories, all nutrients	contains at least 25 percent fewer calories or less of a nutrient than the standard product
light	calories fat sodium	1/3 fewer than the standard product 50 percent less than the standard product 50 percent less than the standard product
less*	calories, nutrients	25 percent less than the standard product
lean	meat, fish, poultry	less than 10 g fat and 0.5 g or less saturated fat and less than 95 mg cholesterol per 100-g serving
extra lean	meat, fish, poultry	less than 5 g fat and less than 2 g saturated fat and less than 95 mg cholesterol per 100-g serving
high	all nutrients	20 percent or more of the % Daily Value per serving
more	all nutrients	at least 10 percent more of a particular % Daily Value than the standard product
good source	all nutrients	10 to 19 percent of the % source Daily Value for a specific nutrient

*"Fewer" is a synonym for "less."

Source: "The new food label," *FDA Backgrounder*, April 1994.

SOURCES

Appell, Glenn D., "Weight control products," *Handbook of Nonprescription Drugs,* 9th ed. (Washington, DC: American Pharmaceutical Association, 1990).

Chrebet, Jennifer, "Diet drugs," *American Health,* April 1995.

Fraser, Laura, "Dieting by prescription," *Vogue,* May 1995.

Food and Drug Administration, Food Safety and Inspection Service, "An introduction to the new food label" (Washington, DC: USDA/DHHS Publication No. [FDA] 94-2271, October 1993).

Long, James W., and James J. Rybacki, *The Essential Guide to Prescription Drugs 1995* (New York: HarperCollins, 1995).

"The new food label," *FDA Backgrounder,* April 1994.

Physicians' Desk Reference, 48th ed. (Montvale, NJ: Medical Economics Data, 1994).

Raloff, J, "Coming: Drug therapy for chocoholics?" *Science News,* June 17, 1995.

Tannen, Mary, "The way of all flesh," *New York Times Magazine,* May 14, 1995.

Travis, J., "Mouse obesity cured by hormone," *Science News,* July 25, 1995.

CHAPTER 6

HOME HEALTH TESTS

As our interest in preventive medicine has grown, so has the market for tests that allow us to monitor our health in the privacy of our own homes.

Home health tests are a real advance in medical care. They give us a relatively inexpensive, relatively simple way to detect early warning signs of potentially serious problems such as colon cancer or urinary infections; to monitor an existing condition such as our cholesterol level; or to predict events such as ovulation and enhance our ability to achieve a goal—pregnancy.

But if home tests are a convenience, they are also a responsibility. Running a medical test requires us to exercise the kind of judicious care we expect from our health professionals. To use home tests safely and successfully, follow these steps:

1. *Read the package label.* All home tests rely on chemical indicators, so it is important not to buy or use a test later than the expiration date printed on the carton. Storage counts, too. If you leave the test in a place where the temperature is too high or too low, that may weaken or inactivate the chemicals and lead to an inaccurate result.

2. *Follow directions to the letter.* Before running any self-test at home, read the package and the package insert carefully. Do not substitute materials. For example, if the test requires you to collect urine, use the container that comes with the kit. Make a checklist of the steps to prepare for the test. Are there any foods or drugs to avoid? Do certain health conditions preclude your using this test? Do you have to prepare any equipment? The time you spend in preparation will pay off in a more accurate test reading. For extra insurance, it is often a good idea to run more than one test.

3. *Discuss the results with your doctor.* No test is perfect. Even when you think you have done everything right, it is still possible to

get a false positive result, suggesting that you have a condition when you do not, or a false negative result, failing to detect a condition that is really present. Professional follow-up makes home testing safer and more reliable.

OVULATION TEST KITS

This test predicts fertility based on the amount of luteinizing hormone in your urine. Luteinizing hormone, also known as LH or lutropin, is secreted by the pituitary gland midway through the menstrual cycle. A rise in the levels of LH triggers the release of a mature egg from an ovarian follicle, the event we call ovulation. Female urine always contains some LH, but the release of the egg is preceded by a clear and detectable hormone surge recognized by the chemicals in ovulation detector kits.

HOW THIS TEST WORKS

Most ovulation tests (ANSWER, CONCEIVE, FIRST RESPONSE, OVUQUICK, Q-TEST) require you to urinate into a small cup and then use a dropper to add a few drops of urine into a test vial, which changes color within 3 to 5 minutes to indicate an LH surge. OVUKIT, a more sensitive test meant primarily for women using fertility drugs, also uses the cup-and-dropper method, but it takes as long as an hour to provide results. CLEARPLAN EASY uses a different method, a test strip you hold in your urine stream for 5 seconds. You can read the results in 5 minutes, and if you wish, you can freeze the test to show the results to your partner (or your doctor) at a later date.

You perform the ovulation test on a day in your menstrual cycle chosen by counting forward from the *first day* (day one) of menstrual bleeding, even if it is only spotting.

Ovulation normally occurs within 12 to 24 hours after the LH surge. Because the egg can be fertilized for only 6 to 24 hours after ovulation, women who wish to become pregnant will have intercourse on the day of the surge. On the other hand, because sperm can survive for at least 72 hours (three days) in the female reproductive tract, women who are using the ovulation predictor test as part of a natural family planning regimen (see pages 103–104) to postpone pregnancy must refrain from intercourse from the start of menstruation to at

WHEN TO USE AN OVULATION TEST KIT	
Counting from the first day of menstrual bleeding	
If your menstrual cycle is	*. . . start testing on*
22 days or fewer	day 7
23 to 32 days	day 11
33 days or longer	day 17

Source: Product insert, ANSWER ovulation test kit, Carter Products division of Carter Wallace, New York 10105 (1990, 1994).

least two days after ovulation occurs. This schedule is comparable to the temperature method plus the mucus method of natural family planning, but more rigorous than the mucus method alone. "The mucus method is a better guide," says Sheila Power Potter, coordinator of the Natural Family Planning Apostolate of the Archdiocese of New York. "It is less expensive and it gives you many more 'safe' days during the month."

IS THIS TEST ACCURATE?

According to their manufacturers, ovulation test kits are accurate 94 percent to 99 percent of the time when run and read by laboratory technicians.

However, a number of variables may lead to an erroneous result. The first is the most obvious: if your cycles are not completely regular, you may not ovulate when you expect to. A shorter-than-normal cycle means you may ovulate before you begin testing; a longer-than-normal cycle means you may ovulate after the tests are done. That's why ovulation test kits are not marketed as a birth control method.

Taking birth control pills will not influence this test, but if you are using the fertility drug clomiphene citrate (CLOMID, SERAPHENE), a nonsteroidal compound that has some chemical properties similar to estrogen, your urine will always produce a light pink result. To pinpoint ovulation, you must repeat the test until the day when the color is significantly darker, indicating the LH surge.

COMPARING THE PRODUCTS: OVULATION TEST KITS

Product (Supplier)	Urine Collection Method	Detection Time	Manufacturer's Estimate of Accuracy in Laboratory Testing	For Assistance
ANSWER (Carter Products)	Cup	3 minutes	99 percent	1-212-339-5000*
CLEARPLAN EASY (Unipath/ Whitehall Laboratories)	Hold test strip in urine stream for 5 seconds	5 minutes[†]	98 percent	1-800-883-EASY
CONCEIVE** (Quidel)	Cup	3 minutes	98.3 percent	1-800-874-1517
FIRST RESPONSE (Carter Products)	Cup	3 minutes	99 percent	1-800-367-6022
OvuKIT[††] (Quidel)	Cup	1 hour	96 percent	1-800-874-1517
OVUQUICK[††] (Quidel)	Cup	4 minutes	94 percent	1-800-874-1517
Q-TEST** (Quidel)	Cup	3 minutes	98.3 percent	1-800-874-1517

* If you are calling long distance, the operator will call you back.

† The first results of this test may be visible in 1 minute, but the manufacturer recommends waiting 5 minutes for conclusive results.

†† These two tests are more expensive and complicated and may take longer than 1-step tests to produce results. They are designed not for family planning but for women who are being treated for infertility.

** Product insert printed in English and Spanish.

Sources: ANSWER, CONCEIVE, FIRST RESPONSE, OvuKIT, OVUQUICK, Q-TEST package inserts. *Physicians' Desk Reference for Nonprescription Drugs*, 16th ed. (Montvale, NJ: Medical Economics Data, 1995).

PREGNANCY TEST KITS

Like ovulation predictor kits, pregnancy tests work by detecting rising levels of a hormone in your urine. The hormone is human chorionic gonadotropin (HCG), secreted by the chorion, a membrane surrounding the fetus in the uterus.

HOW THIS TEST WORKS

The first generation of home pregnancy tests, starting with e.p.t. (introduced in 1977), relied on a process called *hemagglutination inhibition reaction*. In this test, a few drops of urine are added to a vial containing a small amount of red blood cells coated with HCG antigen and anti-serum. If HCG is present in the urine, the hormone will form a complex with the anti-serum; stripped of the HCG antigen, the red blood cells will fall to the bottom of the test tube forming the dough-nut-shaped ring that signifies a positive result: pregnancy.

A pregnant woman's HCG levels double every 1.7 days; they are highest in the "morning urine," the urine that collects in the bladder overnight. Because the original pregnancy test kits required a high level of HCG, they were most accurate early in the morning, in the third or fourth week of pregnancy, approximately 9 days after a missed period. The test could take anywhere from 30 minutes to an hour to get results, and any vibration near the test—a ringing telephone, a humming refrigerator—could produce a false negative or false positive.

Current home pregnancy tests are more sensitive, faster, and more accurate. They use the advanced technology called *monoclonal antibodies,* the same procedure used to detect the HIV virus linked to AIDS. A monoclonal antibody is a substance biologically engineered to react to only one antigen. If there is HCG in your urine, the monoclonal antibody in the test will bind to the HCG. Then the HCG/antibody complex will bind to a second antibody, producing the color change that signifies pregnancy.

Monoclonal antibody pregnancy tests are very sensitive. You can use them morning, noon, or night, on the first day of a missed period (theoretically the fourteenth day of pregnancy). ADVANCE, CONCEIVE, FACT PLUS, Q-TEST, and RAPIDVUE employ the cup method of urine collection. ANSWER, CLEARBLUE EASY, CONFIRM, e.p.t., FIRST RESPONSE, and FORTEL provide a stick to be held in your urine stream.

All show results within three to five minutes. (Note: Home pregnancy tests are not specific for ectopic pregnancy; they may or may not detect this potentially fatal condition.)

IS THIS TEST ACCURATE?

Like ovulation test kits, pregnancy test kits come up with the correct result 98 percent to 99 percent of the time in laboratory testing, that is, when performed and interpreted by a trained technician. As you might expect, consumers are more likely to make a mistake in running the test or reading the results. The results of your pregnancy test will not be affected by birth control pills, the injectable contraceptive Depo-Provera (NORPLANT), the fertility drug clomiphene citrate (CLOMID, SEROPHENE), menopause, menstruation, or a yeast infection. But if you are taking hormones such as HCG, menotropins (PERGONAL), or uro-follitropin (METRODIN) as treatment for infertility, the test will detect the hormones and show a positive result even if you are not pregnant.

If you collect your urine in a cup with a waxed surface rather than the cup that comes in the kit, you may run into the opposite problem. Wax particles from the cup will mix with your urine, clogging the test strip so as to prevent the antibodies from reacting. Even if you are pregnant, the test may read negative.

When you read the test result at the end of the specified time period, if it is negative, do not keep the test around to read again later in the day. The chemicals in the test will continue to react so that after 30 minutes or so a negative result may begin to look weakly positive. On the other hand, a positive result will stay the same for several days, giving you plenty of time to show it to your partner or your doctor.

See the charts below for a comparison of pregnancy test kits.

COMPARING THE PRODUCTS: PREGNANCY TEST KITS

Product (Supplier)	Features
1 STEP ADVANCE (Advanced Care Products/Johnson & Johnson)	**Urine collection method:** Collect urine in cup; use dropper to add urine to test. **Results appear in:** 5 minutes. Two colored lines in "result window" indicate pregnancy. **Manufacturer's estimate of test accuracy:** 99 percent accurate in laboratory testing; 98 percent accurate in consumer testing. **For assistance:** 1-800-526-3979, 8 A.M.–5 P.M. Monday–Friday, Eastern Time
ANSWER* Quick and Simple (Carter Products)	**Urine collection method:** Hold test stick in urine stream for 10 seconds or urinate into cup and dip stick into cup. **Results appear in:** 3 minutes. Pink or purple bar in "result window" indicates pregnancy. **Manufacturer's estimate of test accuracy:** 99+ percent accurate in laboratory testing; 96 to 97 percent accurate in consumer testing. **For assistance:** (212) 339-5000 (If you are calling long distance, they will call you back.)
CLEARBLUE EASY (Unipath/Whitehall Laboratories)	**Urine collection method:** Hold absorbent end of test stick in urine stream. **Results appear in:** 3 minutes. **Manufacturer's estimate of test accuracy:** 99 percent accurate in laboratory testing. **For assistance:** 1-800-883-EASY (1-800-883-3279)
CONCEIVE (Quidel)	**Urine collection method:** Collect urine in cup; use dropper to add urine to test. **Results appear in:** A positive result may appear as quickly as 1 minute, but it is more reliable to wait 3 minutes. A blue "control" line plus a parallel pink-to-purple line indicate pregnancy. If the pink line takes longer than 1 minute to appear, retest in a few days. **Manufacturer's estimate of test accuracy:** 99.5 percent accurate in laboratory testing. **For assistance:** 1-800-266-2348, 7 A.M.– 5 P.M. Pacific Time

Product (Supplier)	Features
CONFIRM 1-STEP (Schmid Laboratories)	**Urine collection method:** Hold absorbent end of stick in urine stream for 5 seconds. **Results appear in:** 5 minutes. Colored bar in heart-shaped window indicates pregnancy. **Manufacturer's estimate of test accuracy:** 99+ percent accurate in laboratory testing. **For assistance:** 1-800-827-0987
e.p.t. Quickstick (Parke Davis)	**Urine collection method:** Hold absorbent end of test stick in urine stream for 5 seconds. **Results appear in:** 2 minutes. Results *must* be read before 20 minutes to avoid inaccuracy due to dye leakage. **Manufacturer's estimate of test accuracy:** 99+ percent accurate in laboratory testing. **For assistance:** 1-800-562-0266
FACT PLUS (Advanced Care Products/Johnson & Johnson)	**Urine collection method:** Urinate into cup. Use dropper to add urine to test. **Results appear in:** 5 minutes. Colored "plus sign" in "result window" indicates pregnancy. **Manufacturer's estimate of test accuracy:** 99 percent accurate in laboratory testing; 98 percent accurate in consumer testing. **For assistance:** 1-800-526-3979, 8 A.M.–5 P.M., Monday–Friday, Eastern Time. Note: The package insert is printed in English and Spanish.
FIRST RESPONSE* 1-STEP (Carter Products)	**Urine collection method:** Hold absorbent end of test stick in urine stream for at least 10 seconds. **Results appear in:** 3 minutes. Pink or purple bar in "result window" indicates pregnancy. **Manufacturer's estimate of test accuracy:** 99+ percent accurate in laboratory testing; 96 to 97 percent accurate in consumer testing. **For assistance:** 1-800-367-6022, 7 A.M.–5 P.M., Monday–Friday, Eastern Time
FORTEL (Biomerica)	**Urine collection method:** Hold absorbent end of test stick in urine stream for at least 10 seconds. **Results appear in:** 5 minutes. Pink band in test window indicates pregnancy. **Manufacturer's estimate of test accuracy:** 99.9 percent accurate in laboratory testing. **For information:** 1-800-854-3002

Product (Supplier)	Features
Q-TEST (Quidel)	**Urine collection method:** Collect urine in cup; use dropper to add urine to test. **Results appear in:** A positive result may appear as quickly as 1 minute, but it is more reliable to wait 3 minutes. A blue "control" line plus a parallel pink-to-purple line indicate pregnancy. **Manufacturer's estimate of test accuracy:** 99.5 percent accurate in laboratory testing. **For assistance:** 1-800-874-1517, 7 A.M.–5 P.M., Pacific Time
RAPIDVUE (Quidel)	**Urine collection method:** Collect urine in cup; use dropper to add urine to test. **Results appear in:** 3 minutes. A blue "control" line plus a parallel pink-to-purple line, however faint, indicate pregnancy; if the pink line appears later than 3 minutes, retest in a few days. **Manufacturer's estimate of test accuracy:** 99.5 percent accurate in laboratory testing. **For assistance:** 1-800-266-2348, 7 A.M.–5 P.M., Monday–Friday, Pacific Standard Time. Note: the package insert is printed in English and Spanish.

*ANSWER and FIRST RESPONSE are both produced by Carter Products Laboratory, a division of Carter Wallace. The only difference between the kits is that FIRST RESPONSE, which is advertised nationally, comes with an 800 number.

Sources: Product inserts for ADVANCE, ANSWER, CONFIRM, e.p.t. Quickstick, FACT PLUS, FIRST RESPONSE, FORTEL, Q-TEST, RAPIDVUE. Whitehall action line (CLEARBLUE EASY). Consumer assistance, Schmid (FACT PLUS).

CHOLESTEROL TESTS

Cholesterol is a fatty substance produced naturally in the liver. We also get cholesterol from the food we eat. Cholesterol circulates in the blood. When the level of cholesterol rises, there is a greater chance that some will stick to the walls of the arteries, narrowing the passages and increasing the risk of heart attack or stroke.

It is easy enough to determine where you sit on the cholesterol scale. All it takes is a simple blood test that measures cholesterol levels in terms of the number of milligrams (mg) of cholesterol per deciliter (dL) of blood.* Based on this, the National Cholesterol Education Program has arbitrarily divided cholesterol test results into three groups: desirable (less than 200 mg/dL), borderline-high (200–239 mg/dL), and high (more than 240 mg/dL).

Despite these labels, experience has shown that some people with low cholesterol levels suffer heart attacks while others with high readings do not. One explanation for this apparent paradox is the fact that cholesterol is not the only risk factor for heart disease. Others include medical conditions (high blood pressure, diabetes, vascular disease), age (older than 45 for a man, older than 55 for a woman), family history (close relatives who suffered heart disease before age 55), and personal habits (smoking, being more than 30 percent overweight, lack of exercise).

In addition, it is not enough simply to know your overall cholesterol level. It is also important to know the ratio of lipoproteins, the fat and protein particles that carry cholesterol through the bloodstream. High-density lipoproteins (HDLs), the so-called "good" cholesterol, are too large to pass through the walls of arteries, so they usually carry cholesterol out of the body. Low-density lipoproteins (LDLs) and very-low-density lipoproteins (VLDLs), the "bad" cholesterol, are smaller. They may pass through artery walls, leaving cholesterol behind to form plaques (deposits) on the inside of the blood vessels.

During the childbearing years, women are less likely than men to have high cholesterol levels. In addition, they are more likely to have favorable ratios of HDLs to LDLs. Both appear to be influenced by the female sex hormone, estrogen. At menopause, as estrogen secretion declines, women's cholesterol levels begin to rise, and levels of HDLs

---

* A deciliter is 1/100th of a liter.

decline. In old age, a woman's risk of heart attack and stroke approaches (but never quite equals) a man's.*

HOW THIS TEST WORKS

ADVANCED CARE CHOLESTEROL TEST, introduced in 1994, is simple and easy to perform. The kit contains a small, sterile lancet with which to puncture the skin on either your middle or "ring" finger. Holding your finger above the test cassette, you spill a few drops of blood into a special well. After 2 to 4 minutes, you activate the test by pulling a tab at the side of the cassette. In approximately 15 minutes, a colored bar appears on a "measurement scale," which looks something like a thermometer. To obtain your total cholesterol level, you compare the bar to a "result chart."

IS THIS TEST ACCURATE?

In consumer studies, ADVANCED CARE delivered an accurate result 97 percent of the time. The most likely explanation for an inaccurate reading, either too high or too low, is failure to follow directions. For example, if you open the package and leave it lying around for a couple of hours or days before using the test, exposure to air may affect the chemicals in the cassette. If you do not drip enough blood into the test well, the reading may be falsely low. After you start the test, the chemicals continue to react, so if you wait longer than 30 minutes to read the result, it may be falsely high. If you run the test in direct sunlight, you may end up with no visible result at all.

You don't have to fast before using this test, as most foods do not interfere with the test results. However, if you have taken more than 500 mg of vitamin C or a standard dose of acetaminophen (TYLENOL) within four hours of taking this test, your cholesterol level will read lower than it really is. If you are taking birth control pills or are pregnant or have been ill recently, the cholesterol reading will be accurate

---

* Estrogen does not lend the same protection to men. In fact, early in the 1970s, when men participating in the well-known Framingham Heart Study were given female hormones in an attempt to lower their risk of heart attack, the result was exactly the opposite of what the researchers had expected. Blood clots and heart attacks increased; the experiment was abandoned. Newer studies suggest that just as estrogen protects women, testosterone protects men.

at the moment you take the test but may not reflect your real, long-term levels.

The drawback to this test is that it gives you only the total cholesterol level; it does not show lipoprotein ratios. In addition, the results may vary as much as 10 to 15 percent between tests depending on a slew of variables including diet and health. In other words, ADVANCED CARE's true value is as a guide, not a diagnosis. For a complete cholesterol reading, along with an evaluation of your personal risk of heart disease or stroke, the final source is still your doctor.

OCCULT FECAL BLOOD TESTS

Colorectal cancer is the third leading cancer and the third leading cause of cancer death among Americans, men as well as women. Women who have had breast cancer or cancer of the genitals have a higher-than-normal risk of colon cancer.

Early detection of colorectal cancer is important to survival. If these tumors are discovered at an early stage while they are still localized, the five-year survival rates are 93 percent for colon cancer and 87 percent for cancer of the rectum. The least invasive test for colon cancer is one that detects occult (hidden) blood in the stool. The American Cancer Society recommends this once a year for everyone age 50 or older.

HOW THIS TEST WORKS

Modern self-tests for occult fecal blood (EZ DETECT, ColoCARE) do not require you to collect a stool sample. Instead, the test contains biodegradable pads impregnated with tetramethylbenzidine, a chemical that turns blue or green in the presence of hemoglobin, the red pigment in blood cells. To perform the test, you simply drop the pad, printed side up, into the toilet bowl after a bowel movement. If there is blood in the bowl, the pad will change color.

IS THIS TEST ACCURATE?

This test is accurate, with limitations—the principal one being that it is not a diagnostic exam for colon cancer.

First, it is designed simply to detect hidden blood in stool. It will find blood deposited on the outer surface of the stool as it passes through the lower portion of the intestinal tract. But it cannot find blood inside a stool sample, which means that it cannot detect bleeding in the upper part of the tract.

Second, intestinal lesions generally bleed intermittently, that is, from time to time. Even if you use all the test pads in the kit, you may be using them at times when an existing lesion is quiescent.

Third, cancers are not the only source of blood in stool. Hemorrhoids, anal fissures, or a hard bowel movement that tears the rectal tissue may all leave traces of blood on stool.

Finally, the results of this test may be affected by what you eat, the medications you are taking, and even the chemicals you use to clean the toilet bowl.

If you choose to use a self-test for blood in stool, the following guidelines, suggested by the manufacturers, may improve your ability to prevent a false positive or a false negative result:

1. Before beginning this test, flush the bowl at least twice to wash away any residue of cleaning products. Toilet bowl cleansers and deodorants containing chlorine bleach or ammonia may interact with the chemicals on the test pad to produce a false positive.

2. Do not use this test while you are menstruating, if you have rectal bleeding due to hemorrhoids or constipation, or if you have a urinary infection (there may be blood cells in your urine), a gastric infection, or a bleeding ulcer.

3. If you are using a prescription drug, check with your doctor before beginning this test. Some prescription drugs, as well as aspirin and some nonsteroidal anti-inflammatory products available without a prescription, may irritate the intestinal lining, causing it to bleed.

4. Do not use iron supplements for two days before running this test. Large amounts of iron may interact with tetramethylbenzidine to produce a false positive. You may also wish to avoid red meat or rare fish or poultry, as well as cruciferous vegetables such as broccoli, cauliflower, cabbage, and horseradish. The active chemical in this test may react with these foods; experts differ as to whether this reaction will occur in healthy people.

5. Do not use a mineral oil laxative before running this test; the oil may inhibit the chemical reaction on the test pad.

6. Avoid vitamin C supplements for two days before running the test. Taking more than 250 mg/day may keep this test from reacting to blood.

7. Eat high-fiber foods such as popcorn, peanuts, bran, whole grain, and fresh vegetables for a day or two before taking the test to speed the passage of food through the intestinal tract so that you may be more likely to find a hidden tumor.

8. Do not drop toilet paper into the bowl before reading the test pad. The test detects blood in the mucus covering the stool, but toilet paper may absorb mucus so that there is not enough left in the water to react with the test chemicals.

Note: The safest and most accurate way to use a test for hidden blood in stool is at your doctor's direction, with his or her advice. Because there are so many possible reasons other than cancer for the presence of blood in stool, a positive result on this test does not provide a diagnosis of colon cancer. It is only a screening device that may suggest a need for further testing. Therefore, it is imperative to discuss the results of this test with your doctor.

The chart on page 200 compares the features of two occult fecal blood test products.

COMPARING THE PRODUCTS:
TESTS FOR OCCULT BLOOD IN STOOL

Product (Supplier)	Features
EZ DETECT (Biomerica)	**Active ingredient:** Tetramethylbenzidine **Where to get this test:** The drugstore **Positive result:** Blue cross **Results appear in:** 2 minutes **To check test accuracy:** After three negative tests, drop chemical powder in bowl. Add test sheet. If blue cross appears, test is valid. **For assistance:** 1-800-854-3002
ColoCARE (Helena)	**Active ingredients:** Tetramethylbenzidine **Where to get this test:** At your doctor's office **Positive result:** Blue or green color in test area of pad **Results appear in:** 30 seconds **To check test accuracy:** Test pad has two small boxes. If test is working correctly, one turns blue or green, the other stays white. Any result other than this suggests test is not working properly. **For assistance:** 1-800-231-5663

Sources: Products on sale in New York City, summer 1995. Help line, Biomerica. Technical assistance, Helena Laboratories.

TESTS FOR BLOOD IN THE URINE

The urine of a healthy individual does not contain blood. If blood is present, it is considered a warning of kidney stones, a tumor, high blood pressure, a kidney infection, or (for men) a prostate tumor or infection.

For women, the most useful aspect of a self-test for blood in the urine is as an indicator of a urinary tract infection.

HOW THIS TEST WORKS

A typical kit like the EZ DETECT kit from Biomerica contains six plastic cups and six test strips. Each plastic test strip has two chemically treated pads at the bottom, one blue, the other cream-colored. To run the test, you collect your urine in a cup, then dip the strip into the liquid and hold it so that the colored pads are completely submerged for 5 to 10 seconds. Then lift out the strip and shake it off over the bowl. The results will appear in 1 minute.

There are three possible outcomes:

1. Neither the cream not the blue pad changes color. The test is NEGATIVE.

2. The blue pad is unchanged, but the cream pad shows blue. The test is POSITIVE.

3. The cream pad is unchanged, but the blue pad is pink. The test is INVALID.

IS THIS TEST ACCURATE?

EZ DETECT is sensitive enough to pick up fewer than three red blood cells in 1/100th of a drop of urine. To reduce the risk of an inaccurate result, follow these steps:

1. Keep the test-strip vial tightly closed to avoid exposure to sunlight and moisture, which can inactivate the test chemicals.

2. Never touch the test pads with your fingers. Doing so may alter their pH (acid/base balance), leading to a false negative or false positive result.

3. Be sure the test pads are completely submerged in urine. If they are not, the test result may be wrong, either false positive or false negative. To prevent a false negative result, avoid excessive doses of vitamin C and fruit juices for two days before running the test.

For assistance when running this test, call 1-800-854-3002.

SOURCES

Cancer Facts and Figures—1995 (Atlanta, GA: American Cancer Society, 1995).

Heart and Stroke Facts, 1994 Statistical Supplement (Dallas, TX: American Heart Association, 1994).

Meyer, Susan Pawlak, "In-home diagnostic tests," *Handbook of Nonprescription Drugs,* 9th ed. (Washington, DC: American Pharmaceutical Association, 1990).

Packages or product inserts for ANSWER, CONCEIVE, FIRST RESPONSE, OvuKIT, OvuQuick, Q-TEST (ovulation tests); ADVANCE, ANSWER, CONFIRM, e.p.t. Quickstick, FACT PLUS, FIRST RESPONSE, FORTEL, Q-TEST, RAPIDVUE (pregnancy tests); ADVANCED CARE (cholesterol test); EZ DETECT, ColoCARE (occult fecal blood tests); EZ DETECT (hidden blood in urine test). Technical assistance: Biomerica, Helena, Whitehall (CLEARBLUE EASY).

Physicians' Desk Reference for Nonprescription Drugs, 16th ed. (Montvale, NJ: Medical Economics Data, 1995).

CHAPTER 7

PRESCRIPTION DRUGS: THEIR EFFECTS ON FEMALE SEXUAL AND REPRODUCTIVE FUNCTIONS

Women are different from men. Our bodies have more fat, less muscle. Our bones are smaller, lighter, and less dense. We menstruate; we get pregnant; we nurse.

As a result, when we take prescription drugs, our concerns may be different from those of men. Will the drug affect our menstrual cycles? Will it affect our libido or make sexual intercourse uncomfortable? Will it affect our ability to become pregnant, to carry a baby safely to term, or to nurse a newborn? This chapter answers those questions for several hundred common (and not-so-common) prescription drugs. Each entry gives information in five categories:

1. *The product.* This is the drug's generic name followed by some of the *brand name(s)* under which it is commonly sold, promoted, or prescribed.

2. *Use.* This tells you what the drug does.

   Analgesics are painkillers.

   Anti-anginal drugs are used to treat the pain of angina pectoris, a form of heart disease.

   Anti-arrhythmic drugs are used to stabilize an irregular heartbeat.

   Anticancer drugs inhibit the growth or spread of tumors and cancer cells.

   Anticonvulsants prevent or reduce the severity of seizures.

   Antidepressants alter brain chemistry to facilitate the uptake of neurotransmitters, chemicals that affect and usually improve mood.

Anti-emetics prevent or reduce the intensity of vomiting.

Anti-infectives destroy bacteria and other pathogens. Antibiotics are antimicrobials; so are antiviral, antifungal, and antiparasitic drugs.

Antifungal agents inhibit the growth of funguses such as athlete's foot.

Antihypertensives are used to treat high blood pressure.

Anti-inflammatory agents alleviate swelling and redness at the site of an external injury, including an allergic reaction.

Antispasmodics reduce or prevent muscle spasms.

Appetite suppressants reduce the feeling of hunger.

Bronchodilators relax and expand the airways; they are used to treat asthma.

Diuretics increase the body's output of fluids.

Fertility drugs induce ovulation.

Immunosuppressants reduce the body's natural response against invaders; they are used most often to reduce the effects of arthritis, an auto-immune disease, or to lessen rejection after transplant procedures.

NSAIDs (nonsteroidal anti-inflammatory drugs) are analgesics that relieve pain and inflammation without many of the side effects associated with steroid hormones.

Tranquilizers affect brain chemistry to relieve anxiety.

3. ***Adverse effects important to women.*** This category includes information about the drug's effect on fertility, menstruation, and sexual functions, as well as data on its effect on other drugs women may be using or its link to other conditions such as migraine, which affect women more often than men. *These are not the only side effects linked to the drug; they are simply the ones that affect women rather than men.*

4. ***Effect on fetus.*** This tells you whether it is safe to use the drug while you are pregnant. The symbols in this category come from the Food and Drug Administration, which has created a system of ranking the safety of drugs for pregnant women.

5. ***(Effect) in breast milk.*** When you take a drug, will your baby take it too? If you are nursing an infant, this is an important

question. This column tells you whether each drug is excreted in breast milk. As with information about effects on the fetus, this is an evolving category. *If you are planning to nurse your child or are already doing so, ask you doctor about the effects on your child of any drug prescribed for you.*

In this column:

"*yes*"   = the drug is excreted in breast milk
"*yes/?*"   = some evidence, not conclusive
"*?*"   = unknown
"*no*"   = the drug is not excreted in breast milk

	FDA USE-IN-PREGNANCY RATINGS
[A]	means that controlled studies of pregnant women show no risk to the fetus.
[B]	means that there is no evidence of risk to human fetuses. It may be that animal studies show risk but human studies do not, *or* it may be that animal studies show no risk and there have been no adequate studies of human beings.
[C]	means that right now the potential benefits of this drug appear to outweigh the risks—but you cannot rule out the possibility of risk. This assessment may be based on conflicting results from animal studies, or there may be no animal studies and no studies of human beings.
[D]	means that studies show that this drug poses a risk to human fetuses, but the potential benefits are still thought to be solid enough to permit the drug to be used, with caution, in serious disease or when a pregnant woman faces a life-threatening situation for which no other drug is considered effective.
[X]	means that the drug should not be used by pregnant women. Animal and human studies show that the risk to the fetus is so great that it outweighs any potential benefits to a pregnant woman who intends to carry her child to term.

NOTE: The FDA rankings in the following drug chart are current as of this writing. However, new studies continually provide additional information about drugs and drug products, which means that the FDA rating may change as more information becomes available. *If you are planning to become pregnant, or if you are already pregnant, check with your doctor when a new drug is prescribed for you.*

PRESCRIPTION DRUGS

Drug (Brand Names)	Use	Adverse Effects Important to Women	Effect on Fetus	In Breast Milk
ACEBUTOLOL (Sectral)	antihypertensive		[B]	yes
ACETAZOLAMIDE (aK-ZOL, Dazamid, Diamox, Storzolamide)	anticonvulsant, antiglaucoma	decreased libido	[C]	yes
ACYCLOVIR (Zovirax)	antiviral	change in menstrual cycle/flow	[C]	?
ALBUTEROL (Proventil, Ventolin)	bronchodilator		[C]	?
ALPRAZOLAM (Xanax)	tranquilizer	inhibited orgasm (rare); change in menstrual cycle/flow	[D]	?
AMANTADINE (Symadine, Symmetrel)	anti-Parkinson's; antiviral		[C]	yes
AMILORIDE (Midamor, Moduretic)	diuretic		[B]	?
AMINOPHYLLINE (Aminophyllin, Phyllocontin, Triphylline)	bronchodilator		[C]	yes
AMITRIPTYLINE (Amatril, Elavil, Endep)	antidepressant	changes in libido; inhibited orgasm; breast enlargement	[C]	yes
AMLODIPINE (Norvasc)	antihypertensive		[C]	?

Drug (Brand Names)	Use	Adverse Effects Important to Women	Effect on Fetus	In Breast Milk
AMOXAPINE (Asendin)	antidepressant	changes in libido; inhibited orgasm; breast enlargement	[C]	yes
AMOXICILLIN (Amoxil, Trimox, Wymox)	antibiotic	reduces the effectiveness of oral contraceptives (rare); breakthrough bleeding may be a sign this is occurring	[B]	yes
AMPICILLIN (Amcill, Omnipen, Polycillin, Principen)	antibiotic		[B]	yes
AZITHOMYCIN (Zithomax)	anti-infective		[B]	?
BACAMPICILLIN (Spectrobid)	antibiotic		[B]	yes
BENAZEPRIL (Lotensin)	antihypertensive		[D]	yes
BETAXOLOL (Betoptic, Kerlone)	antihypertensive	change in menstrual cycle/flow	[C]	yes
BROMOCRIPTINE (Parlodel)	anti-Parkinson's; antilactation	corrects absence of menstruation due to over-production of pituitary hormone	[X]	prevents lactation
BUMETANIDE (Bumex)	diuretic		[C]	?
BUPROPION (Wellbutrin)	antidepressant	changes in menstrual cycle/flow	[B]	yes

Drug (Brand Names)	Use	Adverse Effects Important to Women	Effect on Fetus	In Breast Milk
BUSPIRONE (BuSpar)	tranquilizer	changes in libido; changes in menstrual cycle/flow	[B]	?
CALCITONIN (Calcimar, Cibacalium)	calcium regulator		[C]	yes
CAPTOPRIL (Capoten)	antihypertensive		[D]	yes
CARBAMAZEPINE (Epitol, Tegretol)	anticonvulsant, antineuralgic (relieves nerve pain)	makes oral contraceptives less effective	[C]	yes
CEFACLOR (Ceclor)	antibiotic		[B]	yes
CEFADROXIL (Duricef, Ultracef)	antibiotic		[B]	yes
CEFIXIME (Suprax)	antibiotic		[B]	?
CEFPROZIL (Cefzil)	antibiotic		[B]	?
CEFTRIAXONE (Rocephin)	antibiotic		[B]	yes
CHLORAMBUCIL (Leukeran)	anticancer (leukemia); immuno-suppressant (rheumatoid arthritis)	change in menstrual cycle/flow; infertility due to lack of ovulation	[D]	?
CHLOROQUINE (Aralen)	antimalarial		[C]*	yes

* Experience with this drug prior to creation of the rating system shows deafness, eye damage, and irregular growth in human fetus.

Drug (Brand Names)	Use	Adverse Effects Important to Women	Effect on Fetus	In Breast Milk
CHLORPROPAMIDE (Diabinese)	antidiabetic	water retention; weight gain	[C]	yes
CHLOROTHIAZIDE (Diachlor, Diurigen, Diuril)	diuretic		[C]	yes
CHLORTIANISENE (Tace)	female sex hormone (estrogen)	increased risk of cancer of breast, endometrium, ovary; growth of uterine fibroids; postmenopausal vaginal bleeding; fluid retention; swollen breasts; vaginal secretions; future cancer of vagina/cervix in fetus if taken by pregnant woman	[X]	yes
CHOLESTRYAMINE (Cholybar, Questran)	anticholesterol agent	reduced calcium absorption; increased risk of osteoporosis; change in libido; deficiency in folic acid, a B vitamin that reduces risk of premature delivery and low birthweight	[C]	no
CHORIONIC GONADOTROPIN (Pregnyl, Profasi)	fertility agent; growth hormone	ovarian hyperstimulation syndrome (OHSS); ruptured ovarian cysts; multiple conceptions/births	[C]	n/a

Drug (Brand Names)	Use	Adverse Effects Important to Women	Effect on Fetus	In Breast Milk
CIMETIDINE (Tagamet)*	anti-ulcer		[B]	yes

* In June 1995, FDA approved over-the-counter sale of low-dose cimetidine.

Drug (Brand Names)	Use	Adverse Effects Important to Women	Effect on Fetus	In Breast Milk
CIPROFLOXACIN (Cipro)	anti-infective	migraine; vaginal yeast infections	[C]	yes
CISPLATIN (Platinol)	anticancer (ovarian cancer)	hair loss	[X]	n/a
CLARITHROMYCIN	anti-infective	vaginal yeast infections	[C]	yes
CLINDAMYCIN (Cleocin)	antibiotic	vaginal yeast infections	[B]	yes
CLOMIPHENE (Clomid, Milophene, Serophene)	fertility	ovarian hyperstimulation syndrome (OHSS); enlarged ovaries with abdominal pain; multiple conceptions/births; increased risk of ectopic pregnancy; breast tenderness	*	*

* This fertility drug is never prescribed for women who are pregnant or nursing. If taken inadvertently by a woman who is pregnant, it can cause birth defects in the developing fetus.

Drug (Brand Names)	Use	Adverse Effects Important to Women	Effect on Fetus	In Breast Milk
CLONAZEPAM (Klonopin)	anticonvulsant; anti-anxiety	increased libido	[D]	yes/?
CLONIDINE (Catapres)	antihypertensive	weight gain; decreased libido	[C]	yes
CLOTRIMAZOLE (Lotrimin, Mycelex)	antifungal		[C]	?
CLOXACILLIN (Cloxapen, Tegopen)	antibiotic	vaginal yeast infections	[B]	yes/?

Drug (Brand Names)	Use	Adverse Effects Important to Women	Effect on Fetus	In Breast Milk
CODEINE	painkiller; narcotic		[C]	yes
COLESTIPOL (Colestid)	anticholesterol agent	reduced calcium absorption; increased risk of osteoporosis; change in libido; deficiency in folic acid, a B vitamin that reduces risk of premature delivery and low birthweight	[C]	no
CROMOLYN (Gastrocrom, Nasalcrom)	asthma preventive		[B]	?
CYCLO-PHOSPHAMIDE (Cytoxan, Neosar)	anticancer agent (multiple myeloma, cancer of breast, ovary, leukemia, lymphoma); immuno-suppressant (rheumatoid arthritis, lupus)	change in menstrual cycle/flow; suppressed ovarian function; sterility damage or damage to offspring from genetic damage to eggs	[D]	yes
CYCLOSPORINE (Sandimmune)	immuno-suppressant (in organ transplant, severe psoriasis, Crohn's disease)		[C]	yes
CYTARABINE (Cytosar-U)	anticancer	chromosomal damage/impaired fertility	[D]	?
DACARBAZINE (DTIC-Dome)	anticancer	hair loss	[C]	?
DACTINOMYCIN (Cosmegen)	anticancer	chromosomal damage/impaired fertility	[C]	?

Drug (Brand Names)	Use	Adverse Effects Important to Women	Effect on Fetus	In Breast Milk
DAUNORUBICIN (Cerubidine)	anticancer		[D]	n/a
DESIPRAMINE (Norpramin, Pertofrane)	antidepressant	changes in libido; breast enlargement; milk production	[C]	yes
DEXAMETHASONE (Decadron, Dexasone, Maxidex)	anti-inflammatory	growth of facial hair; change in menstrual cycle/flow	[C]	yes
DIAZEPAM (Valium)	tranquilizer	change in menstrual cycle/ flow; difficulty in achieving orgasm	[D]	yes
DIETHYL-STILBESTROL (DES, Stilphostrol)	female sex hormone (synthetic estrogen)	increased risk of cancer of breast, endometrium, ovary; growth of uterine fibroids; postmenopausal vaginal bleeding; fluid retention; swollen breasts; vaginal secretions; future cancer of vagina/cervix in fetus if taken by pregnant woman	[X]	yes
DIGOXIN (Lanoxin)	heart stimulant		[C]	yes
DILTIAZEM (Cardizem)	anti-angina drug		[C]	yes
DIPHENHYDRA-MINE (Benadryl, Benylin, Compoz, Excedrin P.M., Nytol, Sominex 2)	antihistamine; hypnotic	shorter menstrual cycle	[B]	yes

Drug (Brand Names)	Use	Adverse Effects Important to Women	Effect on Fetus	In Breast Milk
DOXEPIN (Adapin, Sinequan)	antidepressant	enlarged breasts	[C]	yes
DOXORUBICIN (Adriamycin)	anticancer agent (breast cancer)		*	n/a

* Safe use in pregnancy not established

Drug (Brand Names)	Use	Adverse Effects Important to Women	Effect on Fetus	In Breast Milk
DOXYCYCLINE (Vibramycin, Vibra-Tabs)	antibiotic	vaginal yeast infections	[D]	yes
EPINEPHRINE (Adrenalin, Bronkaid Mist, Epipen, Primatene Mist)	anti-asthma; antiglaucoma; decongestant		[C]	yes
EPOETIN (Procrit)	glycoprotein (stimulates growth of red blood cells)		[C]	?
ERGOTAMINE (Ergomar, Ergostat, Wigrettes)	antimigraine	miscarriage	[X]	yes
ERGOTAMINE plus CAFFEINE (Bellergal-S, Cafergot, Ercaf, Wigraine)	antimigraine	miscarriage	[X]	yes
ERYTHROMYCIN (E-Mycin, Ilosone, Robimycin, Wyamycin E)	antibiotic	vaginal yeast infections	[B]	yes

Drug (Brand Names)	Use	Adverse Effects Important to Women	Effect on Fetus	In Breast Milk
ESTRADIOL (Emcyt, Estrace, Estraderm)	female sex hormone	increased risk of cancer of breast, endometrium, ovary; growth of uterine fibroids; postmenopausal vaginal bleeding; fluid retention; swollen breasts; vaginal secretions; future cancer of vagina/cervix in fetus if taken by pregnant woman	[X]	yes
ESTROGENS see Chlorotrianisene; Diethystilbestrol; Estradiol; Estrogens, conjugated; Estrogens, esterfied; Estrone; Estropipate; Ethinyl estradiol; Quinestrol				
ESTROGENS, CONJUGATED (PMB 200, PMB 400, Premarin)	female sex hormone (estrogen)	increased risk of cancer of breast, endometrium, ovary; growth of uterine fibroids; postmenopausal vaginal bleeding; fluid retention; swollen breasts; vaginal secretions; future cancer of vagina/cervix in fetus if taken by pregnant woman	[X]	yes

Drug (Brand Names)	Use	Adverse Effects Important to Women	Effect on Fetus	In Breast Milk
ESTROGENS, ESTERFIED (Estratab, Estratest, Menest)	female sex hormone (estrogen)	increased risk of cancer of breast, endometrium, ovary; growth of uterine fibroids; postmenopausal vaginal bleeding; fluid retention; swollen breasts; vaginal secretions; future cancer of vagina/cervix in fetus if taken by pregnant woman	[X]	yes
ESTRONE (Ogen)	female sex hormone (estrogen) patches	increased risk of cancer of breast, endometrium, ovary; growth of uterine fibroids; postmenopausal vaginal bleeding; fluid retention; swollen breasts; vaginal secretions; future cancer of vagina/cervix in fetus if taken by pregnant woman	[X]	yes
ESTROPIPATE (Ogen, Ortho-Est)	female sex hormone	increased risk of cancer of breast, endometrium, ovary; growth of uterine fibroids; postmenopausal vaginal bleeding; fluid retention; swollen breasts; vaginal secretions; future cancer of vagina/cervix in fetus if taken by pregnant woman	[X]	yes

Drug (Brand Names)	Use	Adverse Effects Important to Women	Effect on Fetus	In Breast Milk
ETHINYL ESTRADIOL PLUS PROGESTINS (Brevicon 21-Day, 28-Day; Demulen 1/35-21, -28, 1/50-21, -28; LevLen 21, 28; Loestrin FE 1/20, 1.5/30; Loestrin 21 1/20, 1/30; Lo/Ovral, Lo/Ovral 28; Modicon 21, 28; Nordette-21, -28; Norinyl 1+35, -21, -28; OrthoCept; OrthoCyclen; OrthoNovum 1/35-21, -28, 7/7/7/21, -28, 10/11-21, -28; Ortho TriCyclen; Ovcon 35, 50; Ovral, Ovral-28; Tri-Levlen 21, 28; Tri-Norinyl 21, 28; Tri-Phasil 21, 28	oral contraceptives	growth of uterine fibroids; increased risk of breast cancer in very young women; change in menstrual patterns (spotting at midcycle); increased risk of vaginal yeast infection; increased risk of migraine; enlarged/tender breasts; later infertility	[X]	yes
ETHOSUXIMIDE (Zarontin)	anticonvulsant	growth of facial hair; vaginal bleeding	[C]	yes
ETOPOSIDE (VePesid)	anticancer	causes chromosomal damage, may impair fertility	[D]	?
ETRETINATE (Tegison)	antipsoriatic	change in menstrual cycle/flow	[X]	?
FAMOTIDINE (Pepcid)	anti-ulcer	decreased libido	[C]	yes

Drug (Brand Names)	Use	Adverse Effects Important to Women	Effect on Fetus	In Breast Milk
FAMCYCLOVIR (Famvir)	antiviral (herpes zoster/shingles)		[B]	?
FLOXURIDINE (FUDR)	anticancer	reduced fertility (in animal studies)	[D]	?
FLUCONAZOLE (Diflucan)	antifungal	may slow the metabolism of the hormones	[C]	yes
FLUCYTOSINE (Ancobon)	antifungal		[C]	?
FLUOXETINE (Prozac)	antidepressant	hair loss (rare); inhibited orgasm	[B]	?
FLURAZEPAM (Dalmane, Durapam)	hypnotic		[X]	yes
FOSINOPRIL (Monopril)	antihypertensive	decreased libido (rare)	[D]	yes
FUROSEMIDE (Lasix)	diuretic, antihypertensive		[C]	yes
GENFIBROZIL (Lopid)	anticholesterol	decreased libido	[B]	?
GLIPIZIDE (Glucotrol)	antidiabetic	fluid retention, weight gain	[C]	?
GLYBURIDE (DiaBeta, Micronase)	antidiabetic		[B]	?
GRISEOFULVIN (Fulvacin P/G, Fulvacin U/F, Grifulvin V, Grisactin, Gris-PEG)	antifungal	makes oral contraceptives less effective	[C]	?
GUANFACINE (Tenex)	antihypertensive		[B]	yes

Drug (Brand Names)	Use	Adverse Effects Important to Women	Effect on Fetus	In Breast Milk
HISTAMINE (H-2) BLOCKING DRUGS *See* Cimetidine; Famotidine; Nizatidine; Ranitidine				
HYDRALAZINE (Alazine, Apresoline)	antihypertensive	water retention	[C]	yes
HYDRALAZINE with hydro-chlorothiazide (also listed)	antihypertensive plus diuretic		[C]	yes
HYDRALAZINE with reserpine	antihypertensive		[C]	yes
HYDROCHLORO-THIAZIDE (Esidrix, HydroDIURIL, Oretic, Thiuretic, Zide)	diuretic	decreased libido	[D]	yes
HYDROCODONE (Hycodan)	analgesic, narcotic		[C]	?
HYDROXY-CHLOROQUINE (Placquenil)	antimalarial, lupus suppressant		[D]	yes
IBUPROFEN (Advil, Motrin, Motrin IB, Nuprin, Rufen)	analgesic, anti-inflammatory	fluid retention, weight gain; excessive menstrual bleeding	[B]	yes
INDAPAMIDE (Lozol)	antihypertensive	decreased libido	[B]	?

Drug (Brand Names)	Use	Adverse Effects Important to Women	Effect on Fetus	In Breast Milk
INDOMETHACIN (Indameth, Indocin)	analgesic, anti-inflammatory (NSAID)	temporary hair loss; fluid retention	[C], [D]*	yes

* This drug is not considered safe for use during the last trimester of pregnancy.

Drug (Brand Names)	Use	Adverse Effects Important to Women	Effect on Fetus	In Breast Milk
INDOQUINOL (Diquinol, Yodoxin)	antiprotozoal		[C]	?
IPROTROPIUM (Atrovent)	bronchodilator		[B]	yes/?
ISONIAZID (Laniazid, Nydrazid, Rifamate, Teebaconin)	antitubercular		[C]	yes
ISOTRETINOIN (Accutane)	anti-acne	decreased libido, decreased vaginal secretions, change in menstrual cycle/flow, breast discharge (rare)	[X]	?
KETOCONAZOLE (Nizoral)	antifungal	change in menstrual cycle/flow	[C]	yes
KETOPROFEN (Orudis)	analgesic, anti-inflammatory (NSAID)	change in menstrual cycle; excessive menstrual bleeding; decreased libido	[B]	yes
KETOROLAC (Acular, Torolac)	analgesic, anti-inflammatory (NSAID)	fluid retention; weight gain	[C]	yes
LABETALOL (Normodyne, Normoside, Trandate)	antihypertensive	decreased vaginal secretions; inhibited orgasm	[C]	yes

Drug (Brand Names)	Use	Adverse Effects Important to Women	Effect on Fetus	In Breast Milk
LEVODOPA (Dopar, Larodopa, Prolopa, Sinemet)	anti-Parkinson's	increased libido	[C]	yes
LEVONORGESTREL (Norplant)	contraceptve (female sex hormones, progestin)	changes in menstrual cycle/flow; midcycle bleeding; increased risk of ectopic pregnancy	[X]	yes
LEVOTHYROXINE (Levothroid, Levoxine, Syroxine, Synthroid)	thyroid hormones	changes in menstrual cycle/flow while adjusting dosages	[A]	yes
LEVOTHYROXINE plus LIOTHYRONINE (Euthroid, Thyrolar)	thyroid hormones	changes in menstrual cycle/flow while adjusting dosages	[A]	yes
LIDOCAINE and PRILOCAINE (Emla cream)	local anesthetic cream		[B]	yes
LIOTHYRONINE (Cytomel, Thyrar)	thyroid hormones	changes in menstrual cycle/flow while adjusting dosages	[A]	yes
LISINOPRIL (Prinivil, Prinzide, Zestoretic, Zestril)	antihypertensive	decreased libido; worsening of lupus	[C]	?
LITHIUM (Cibalith-S, Eskalith, Lithane, Lithobid, Lithonate, Lithotabs)	antidepressant, antimanic mood stabilizer	decreased libido; breast swelling; milk production; weight gain	[D]	yes

Drug (Brand Names)	Use	Adverse Effects Important to Women	Effect on Fetus	In Breast Milk
LOMEFLOXACIN (Maxaquin)	anti-infective	vaginal yeast infections; bleeding between menstrual periods	[C]	yes
LOMUSTINE (CeeNU)	anticancer (brain tumors, Hodgkin's disease)		[D]	
LOPERAMIDE (Imodium, Imodium AD, Pepto Diarrhea Control)	antidiarrheal		[B]	?
LORAZEPAM (Ativan, Lorazepam, Intensol)	tranquilizer		[D]	yes
LOVASTATIN (Mevacor)	anticholesterol		[X]	yes
MAPROTILINE (Ludiomil)	antidepressant	decreased libido; enlarged breasts; milk production	[B]	yes
MECLOFENAMATE (Meclomen)	analgesic (NSAID)	fluid retention	[B], [D]*	yes

    * This drug is not considered safe for use during the last trimester of pregnancy.

MEDROXY-PROGESTERONE (Amen, Curretab, Cycrin, Depo-Provera, Provera)	female sex hormones (progestin)	excessive hair growth; change in menstrual cycle/flow; breast tenderness and secretions; decreased vaginal secretions	[D]	yes
MEFENAMIC ACID (Ponstel)	analgesic (NSAID)		[C]	yes

Drug (Brand Names)	Use	Adverse Effects Important to Women	Effect on Fetus	In Breast Milk
MEGESTROL (Megace)	female sex hormones (progestin)	excessive hair growth; change in menstrual cycle/flow; breast tenderness and secretions; decreased vaginal secretions	[D]	yes
MENOTROPINS (Pergonal)	fertility	ovarian hyperstimulation syndrome (OHSS); enlarged ovaries with abdominal pain; multiple conceptions/births; increased risk of ectopic pregnancy; breast tenderness	[X]	?
MEPERIDINE (Demerol, Pethadol)	analgesic, opiod		[C]	yes
MERCAPTOPURINE (Purinethol)	anticancer (leukemia); immuno-suppressant	cessation of menstruation	[D]	?
MESALAMINE (Asacol, Rowasa)	intestinal anti-inflammatory		[B]	?
MESTRANOL plus PROGESTIN (Norinyl 1+50 -21, -28; Ortho-Novum 1/50-21, -28)	oral contraceptive (female sex hormones)	increased risk of cancer of breast, endometrium, ovary; growth of uterine fibroids; postmenopausal vaginal bleeding; fluid retention; swollen breasts; vaginal secretions; risk of future cancer of vagina/cervix in fetus if taken by pregnant woman	[X]	yes

Drug (Brand Names)	Use	Adverse Effects Important to Women	Effect on Fetus	In Breast Milk
METAPROLOL (Lopressor, Toprol)	antihypertensive	decreased libido; fluid retention; increases effects of oral contraceptives	[C]	yes
META-PROTERENOL (Alupent, Metaprel, Prometa)	bronchodilator	may activate latent diabetes	[C]	?
METHADONE (Dolophine)	analgesic, opiod	decreased libido; inhibited orgasm; lack of menstru-ation (all with long-term use only)	[C]	yes
METHOTREXATE (Folex, Mexate)	anticancer; antipsoriatic	change in menstrual cycle/flow	[X]	yes
METHYLPHENI-DATE (Ritalin)	stimulant		[B]	?
METHYL-PREDNISOLONE (Medrol)	anti-inflammatory, immuno-suppressant		[X]	yes
METHYSERGIDE (Sansert)	antimigraine	fluid retention; weight gain		
METOCLO-PRAMIDE (Maxolon, Octamide, Reglan)	anti-emetic	swollen, tender breasts; milk production; decreased libido; change in menstrual cycle/flow	[B]	yes

Drug (Brand Names)	Use	Adverse Effects Important to Women	Effect on Fetus	In Breast Milk
METRONIDAZOLE (Femazole, Flagyl, Metizol, MetroGel, Metryl, Protostat)	anti-infective	vaginal yeast infection; decreased libido and vaginal secretions	[B]	yes
MINOXIDIL (Loniten, Minodyl, Rogaine)	antihypertensive	excessive growth of body and facial hair; fluid retention, weight gain	[C]	yes
MISOPROSTOL (Cytotec)	ulcer preventive	miscarriage; incomplete abortion with severe uterine bleeding; menstrual irregularity/ cramps; vaginal bleeding between periods/post-menopause	[X]	?
MORPHINE (Astramorph, Duramorph, MS Contin, MSIR, Oramorph, Roxanol)	analgesic, opiod	facial flushing; decreased libido	[C]	yes
NABUMETONE (Relafen)	anti-inflammatory (NSAID)	fluid retention	[B]	yes
NADOLOL (Corgard, Corzide, Apo-Nadol, Syn-Nadol)	anti-anginal, antihypertensive	decreased libido	[C]	yes

Drug (Brand Names)	Use	Adverse Effects Important to Women	Effect on Fetus	In Breast Milk
NAFARELIN (Synarel)	gonadotropin-releasing hormone (relieves symptoms of endometriosis)	estrogen deficiency; masculinizing effects (during treatment); increased loss of bone density (long-term use); decreased libido; decreased vaginal secretions; reduction in breast size	[X]	?
NAPROXEN (Aleve, Anaprox, Naprosyn)	analgesic, anti-inflammatory (NSAID)	fluid retention; weight gain; change in menstrual cycle/flow	[B]	yes
NEDOCROMIL (Tilade)	asthma preventive		[B]	?
NIACIN (Nia-Bid, Niac, Nicobid, Nicolar, Nicotinex)	anticholesterol		[C]	?
NICARDIPINE (Cardene)	anti-anginal, antihypertensive	water retention, ankle swelling; flushing resembling hot flashes	[C]	yes
NICOTINE GUM (Nicorette)	antismoking aid	increased risk of miscarriage	[X]	yes
NICOTINE PATCH (Habitrol, Nicoderm, Nicotrol)	antismoking aid	increased risk of miscarriage	[D]	yes
NIFEDIPINE (Adalat, Procardia)	anti-anginal, antihypertensive	change in menstrual cycle; excessive menstrual bleeding	[C]	?

Drug (Brand Names)	Use	Adverse Effects Important to Women	Effect on Fetus	In Breast Milk
NITROFURANTOIN (Furadantin, Furalan, Furanit, Macrodantin)	urinary antiseptic		[C]	yes
NITROGLYCERIN (Deponit, Minitran, Nitro-Bid, Nitro-cap TD, Nitrocine, Nitrodisc, Nitro-Dur, Nitrogard, Nitroglyn, Nitrol, Nitrong, Nitrostat, Transderm-Nitro)	anti-anginal		[C]	?
NIZATIDINE (Axid)	anti-ulcer	decreased libido	[C]	yes
NORETHINDRONE (Micronor, Nor-Q D)	oral contraceptive (synthetic progestin), "mini-pill"	midcycle menstrual spotting (breakthrough bleeding); less effective than estrogen/progestin combination pill	[X]	yes
NORFLOXACIN (Noroxin)	urinary, ocular anti-infective	depression	[C]	?
NORGESTREL (Ovrette)	oral contraceptive (synthetic progestin), "mini-pill"	less effective than estrogen/progestin combination pill	[X]	yes
NORTRIPTYLINE (Aventyl, Pamelor)	antidepressant	decreased libido; inhibited orgasm; breast enlargement and milk production	[D]	yes

Drug (Brand Names)	Use	Adverse Effects Important to Women	Effect on Fetus	In Breast Milk
OFLOXACIN (Floxin)	anti-infective (urinary, reproductive tract, eyes, and respiratory tract)	vaginitis; painful menstruation; excessive menstrual bleeding	[C]	yes
OLSALAZINE (Dipentium)	anti-inflammatory (bowel)	depression; excessive menstrual bleeding	[C]	?
OMEPRAZOLE (Prilosec)	anti-ulcer	urinary tract infection (rare)	[C]	?
ONDANSETRON (Zofran)	anti-emetic		[B]	*

* Excreted in rats' milk; no studies available for human beings

Drug (Brand Names)	Use	Adverse Effects Important to Women	Effect on Fetus	In Breast Milk
ORAL CONTRACEPTIVES *see* Ethinyl estradiol; Levonorgestrel; Mestranol; Norgestrel; Quinestrol				
OXAPROZIN (Daypro)	analgesic, anti-inflammatory (NSAID)		[C]	yes
OXTRIPHYLLINE (Choledyl)	bronchodilator		[C]	yes
OXYCODONE (Percocet, Percodan, Roxicodone)	analgesic, narcotic		[C]	?
PENBUTOLOL (Levatol)	antihypertensive	decreased libido	[C]	?

Drug (Brand Names)	Use	Adverse Effects Important to Women	Effect on Fetus	In Breast Milk
PENICILLIN V (Beepen VK, Betapen VK, Ledercillin VK, Penapar VK, Pen-Vee K, Robicillin VK, SK-Penicillin VK, Uticillin VK, Veetids)	antibiotic	yeast infections; makes oral contraceptives less effective (rare); breakthrough bleeding may show this is occurring	[B]	yes
PENTAMIDINE (NebuPent)	anti-infective (AIDS-related pneumonia)		[C]	?
PENTAZOCINE (Talacen, Talwin)	analgesic, narcotic		[C], [D]*	?

* In high dose or extended use

Drug (Brand Names)	Use	Adverse Effects Important to Women	Effect on Fetus	In Breast Milk
PERPHENAZINE (Elavil Plus, Etrafon, Levazine, Triavil, Trilafon)	strong tranquilizer	change in menstrual cycle/flow; breast enlargement; milk production; false positive pregnancy test; not for use by breast cancer patients	[C]	yes
PHENELZINE (Nardil)	antidepressant	decreased libido; inhibited orgasm	[C]	yes/?
PHENOBARBITAL (Barbita, Luminal, Solfoton)	sedative, anticonvulsant	decreased libido; makes oral contraceptives less effective	[D]	yes
PHENYTOIN (Dilantin, Diphenylan)	anticonvulsant	excessive growth of body hair; decreased libido; makes oral contraceptives less effective	[D]	yes

Drug (Brand Names)	Use	Adverse Effects Important to Women	Effect on Fetus	In Breast Milk
PILOCARPINE (Almocarpine, Akarpine, Isopto Carpine, Pilagan, Pilocar, Piloptic-1,-2)	antiglaucoma		[C]	?
PINDOLOL (Visken)	antihypertensive	fluid retention; decreased libido; effects of this drug increased by oral contraceptives	[B]	yes
PIRBUTEROL (Maxair)	bronchodilator		[C]	?
PIROXICAM (Feldene)	analgesic, anti-inflammatory (NSAID)	fluid retention (mild); weight gain	[B], [D]*	?

    * This drug is not considered safe for use during the last trimester of pregnancy.

Drug (Brand Names)	Use	Adverse Effects Important to Women	Effect on Fetus	In Breast Milk
PRAVASTATIN (Pravachol)	anticholesterol		[X]	yes
PRAZOSIN (Apro-Prazo, Minipress, Novo-Prazin, Nu-Prazo)	anticholesterol	decreased libido	[C]	yes
PREDNISONE (Deltasone, Meticorten, Orasone, Steraped)	anti-inflammatory	growth of facial hair; water retention; weight gain; change in menstrual cycle/flow	[C]	yes
PRIMAQUINE	antimalarial; anti-infective (AIDS-related pneumonia)		[C]	?

Drug (Brand Names)	Use	Adverse Effects Important to Women	Effect on Fetus	In Breast Milk
PRIMIDONE (Myidone, Mysoline, PMS-Primidone)	anticonvulsant	decreased libido; makes oral contraceptives less effective	[D]	yes
PROBUCOL (Lorelco)	anticholesterol	change in menstrual cycle/flow; rise in blood levels of uric acid	[B]	?
PROCARBAZINE (Matulane)	anticancer		[D]	?
PROCAINAMIDE (Apo-Procainamide, Procainamide SR, Procan SR, Pronestyl)	anti-arrhythmic		[C]	?
PROCHLOR-PERAZINE (Compazine)	strong tranquilizer	change in menstrual cycle/flow; breast enlargement; milk production; false positive pregnancy test; not for use by breast cancer patients	[C]	yes
PROPRANALOL (Inderal, Inderide, Ipran)	anti-anginal, anti-arrhythmic, antihypertensive	decreased libido	[C]	yes
PROTRIPTYLINE (Vivactil)	antidepressant	decreased libido; inhibited orgasm; breast enlargement and milk production	[B]	yes
PYRAZINAMIDE	antituberculosis		[C]	yes

Drug (Brand Names)	Use	Adverse Effects Important to Women	Effect on Fetus	In Breast Milk
PYRIMETHAMINE (Daraprim, Fansidar)	anti-infective (AIDS-related toxoplasmosis, drug-resistant malaria)	folic acid deficiency (increases risk of premature or low-birthweight infant)	[C]	yes
QUAZEPAM (Doral)	hypnotic	decreased libido; oral contra-ceptives increase the sedative effects of this drug	[X]	yes
QUINACRINE (Atabrine)	antiprotozoal; lupus suppressant		[C]	yes
QUINAPRIL (Accupril)	antihypertensive		[C], [D]*	?

* This drug is not considered safe for use during the second and third trimesters of pregnancy.

Drug (Brand Names)	Use	Adverse Effects Important to Women	Effect on Fetus	In Breast Milk
QUINESTROL (Estrovis)	female sex hormone	increased risk of cancer of breast, endometrium, ovary; growth of uterine fibroids; postmenopausal vaginal bleeding; fluid retention; swollen breasts; vaginal secretions; future cancer of vagina/cervix in fetus if taken by pregnant woman	[X]	yes
QUINIDINE (Cardioquin, Cin-Qum, Duraquin, Quinaglute, Quinora)	anti-arrhythmic		[C]	yes

Drug (Brand Names)	Use	Adverse Effects Important to Women	Effect on Fetus	In Breast Milk
RAMIPRIL (Altace)	antihypertensive		[D]*	yes
* This drug is not considered safe for use during the second and third trimesters of pregnancy.				
RANITIDINE (Zantac)	anti-ulcer	decreased libido	[B]	yes
RIFABUTIN (Mycobutin)	antimycobacterial (AIDS-related mycobacterium avium complex [MAC])	change in menstrual cycle/ flow; makes oral contraceptives less effective	[B]	?
RIFAMPIN (Rifadin, Rifamate, Rimactane)	antibiotic	change in menstrual cycle/ flow; makes oral contraceptives less effective	[C]	yes
RISPERIDONE (Risperdal)	antipsychotic (schizophrenia resistent to other drugs)	increased secretion of prolactin; breast tenderness and swelling	[C]	yes
SALMETEROL (Serevent)	anti-asthma		[C]	yes
SERTRALINE (Zoloft)	antidepressant	inhibited orgasm	[B]	?
SIMVASTATIN (Zocor)	anticholesterol		[X]	?
SPIRONO-LACTONE (Alatone, Aldactazide, Aldactone)	diuretic	hair growth; deepening voice; decreased libido; breast enlarge-ment; vaginal bleeding; decreased vaginal secretions	[D]	yes*
* A chemical produced by the metabolism of this drug is present in breast milk				

Drug (Brand Names)	Use	Adverse Effects Important to Women	Effect on Fetus	In Breast Milk
STAVUDINE (Zerit)	antiviral (AIDS)		[C]	yes
SUCRALFATE (Carafate)	anti-ulcer drug		[B]	?
SULFADIAZINE (Microsulfon, Trisem, Trisoralem)	anti-infective		[C]	yes
SULFAMETH-OXAZOLE (Gantanol and several combin-ation drugs)	anti-infective		[C]	yes
SULFASALAZINE (Azaline, Azulfidine, SAS-500)	anti-inflammatory (bowel)		[B]	yes
SULFISOXAZOLE (Gantrisin, Lipo Gantrisin, SK-Soxazole)	anti-infective		[C]	yes
SULINDAC (Clinoril)	analgesic, anti-inflammatory	enlarged breasts; endometrial bleeding	[D]	?*

  * This drug is not considered safe for use during the third trimester of pregnancy.

Drug (Brand Names)	Use	Adverse Effects Important to Women	Effect on Fetus	In Breast Milk
SUMATRIPTAN (Imitrex)	antimigraine		[C]	?*

  * Sumatriptan is excreted in breast milk of animals; no data on human beings available

Drug (Brand Names)	Use	Adverse Effects Important to Women	Effect on Fetus	In Breast Milk
TAMOXIFEN (Nolvadex)	anti-estrogen; anti-cancer	increased risk of endometrial cancer; change in menstrual cycle/flow; postmenopausal vaginal bleeding; fluid retention, weight gain; effectiveness reduced by estrogens/oral contraceptives	[D]	?
TERAZOSIN (Hytrin)	antihypertensive	fluid retention; oral contraceptives make this drug less effective	[C]	?
TERBUTALINE (Brethaire, Brethine, Bricanyl)	anti-asthmatic; bronchodilator		[B]	yes
TERFENADINE (Seldane)	antihistamine	change in menstrual cycle/flow; enlarged breasts; milk production	[C]	?
TETRACYCLINE (Achromycin, Actisite, Cyclopar, Mysteclin-F, Nova-Tetra, Nor-Tex, Panmycin, Robitet, Sumycin, Tetra-C, Tetracyn, Tetralen, Tetram, Topicycline)	antibiotic	vaginal yeast infections; makes oral contraceptives less effective	[D]	yes

Drug (Brand Names)	Use	Adverse Effects Important to Women	Effect on Fetus	In Breast Milk
THEOPHYLLINE (Accurbron Bronkodyl, Constant-T, Elixicon, Elixophyllin, Lodrane, Lodrane CR, Respid, Slo-bid, Slo-Phyllin, Sustaire, Theobid Dura-caps, Theochron, Theo-Dur, Theolair, Theophyl-SR, Theo-24, Theovent, Theox)	anti-asthmatic, bronchodilator	oral contraceptives make theophylline stronger	[C]	yes
THIORIDAZINE (Mellaril, Millazine)	tranquilizer (strong)	decreased libido; inhibited orgasm; change in menstrual cycle/flow; enlarged breasts; false positive pregnancy test results; not for use by breast cancer patients	[C]	yes
THIOTHIXENE (Navane)	tranquilizer (strong)	change in menstrual cycle/flow; breast enlargement; milk production; false positive pregnancy test; not for use by breast cancer patients	[C]	?
TIMOLOL (Blocadren, Timoptic)	anti-anginal, antihypertensive, antimigraine	decreased libido	[C]	yes
TOLAZAMIDE (Ronase, Tolamide, Tolinase)	antidiabetic		[C]	yes

Drug (Brand Names)	Use	Adverse Effects Important to Women	Effect on Fetus	In Breast Milk
TOLBUTAMIDE (Oramide, Orinase)	antidiabetic		[C]	yes
TOLMETIN (Tolectin)	analgesic, anti-inflammatory (NSAID)		[B]	?
TRAZODONE (Desyrel, Trialodine)	antidepressant	increased libido; change in menstrual cycle/flow	[C]	yes
TRIAMCINOLONE (Aristocort, Azmacort, Kenacort, Nasacort)	anti-asthmatic	osteoporosis (long-term use)	[C]	?
TRIAMTERENE (Dyrenium)	antidiabetic		[B]	yes
TRIFLUOPERAZINE (Stelazine, Suprezine)	tranquilizer, antipsychotic	change in menstrual cycle/flow; enlarged breasts; delayed orgasm; not for use by breast cancer patients	[C]	yes
TRIMETHOPRIM PLUS SULFA-METHOXAZOLE (Bactrim, Betha-prim, Comoxol, Cotrim, Proloprim, Septra, Sulfaprim D/S, Trimpex, Uroplus DS)	urinary anti-infective		[C]	yes

Drug (Brand Names)	Use	Adverse Effects Important to Women	Effect on Fetus	In Breast Milk
UROFALLITOPIN (Metrodin)	fertility drug	ovarian hyperstimulation syndrome (OHSS); enlarged ovaries with abdominal pain; multiple conceptions/births; increased risk of ectopic pregnancy; breast tenderness	[X]	?
VALPROIC ACID (Depa, Depakene, Depakote, Deproic)	anticonvulsant	change in menstrual cycle/flow; enlarged breasts; decreased libido; makes oral contraceptives less effective	[D]	yes
VANCOMYCIN (Vancocin)	antibiotic		[B]	yes
VENLAFAXINE (Effexor)	antidepressant		[C]	?
VERAPAMIL (Calan, Isoptin, Verelan)	anti-anginal, anti-arrhythmic, antihypertensive	fluid retention, change in menstrual cycle/flow	[C]	yes
VINBLASTINE (Velban)	anticancer (Hodgkin's disease, choriocarcinoma, breast cancer)		[D]	?
VINCRISTINE (Oncovin)	anticancer (Hodgkin's disease, lymphoma)	amenorrhea	[D]	?

Drug (Brand Names)	Use	Adverse Effects Important to Women	Effect on Fetus	In Breast Milk
WARFARIN (Carfin, Coumadin, Panwarfin, Sofarin)	anticoagulant		[X]	yes
ZALCITABINE (HIVID)	antiviral (HIV)		[C]	?
ZIDOVUDINE (Retrovir)	antiviral (HIV)		[C]	?
ZOLPIDEN (Ambien)	hypnotic		[B]	yes

SOURCES

Chemotherapy and You, NIH Publication No. 88–1136 (Bethesda, MD: National Cancer Institute, 1988).

Long, James W., and James J. Rybacki, *The Essential Guide to Prescription Drugs 1995* (New York: HarperCollins, 1995).

The Merck Manual, 16th ed. (Rahway, NJ: Merck, Research Laboratories, 1992).

The Merck Manual of Geriatrics (Rahway, NJ: Merck, Sharpe and Dohme Research Laboratory, 1990).

National Research Council, *Recommended Dietary Allowances*, 10th ed. (Washington, DC: National Academy Press, 1989).

Physicians' Desk Reference, 48th ed. (Montvale, NJ: Medical Economics Data, 1994).

Schein, Jeff, "A prescription for trouble: When medications don't mix," *Priorities,* 7, no. 2, 1995.

INGREDIENTS AND LABEL TERMS
FOR NONPRESCRIPTION DRUGS AND
OTHER OVER-THE-COUNTER PRODUCTS

Some ingredients in over-the-counter (OTC) products have more than one chemical or trade name. In this glossary, synonyms are listed in parentheses following the ingredient name:

Gum arabic (*Acacia*)

Closely related ingredients, which do the same job and may cause the same side effects, are listed this way:

Zinc undecylenate. See Undecylenic acid.

Some words used in definitions also have their own separate listing in the glossary. These terms are followed with "*(gl.)*", as in:

Maltodextrin. A texturizer *(gl.)* and flavor enhancer created from cornstarch. Used to "bulk up" liquid diet formula foods.

The fact that some ingredients in this glossary are described as being allergenic, irritating, or toxic to some people in some specific situations may not mean that they will be allergenic, irritating, or toxic to everybody all the time. Finally, having an irritating or toxic ingredient in a product does not necessarily mean that the product itself is either irritating or toxic; the effects attributed to the concentrated, isolated ingredient may differ markedly from the effects of a product containing a more dilute concentration of the offending ingredient.

A

Absorbency. The amount of liquid a substance can draw in and hold.
Following the emergence of toxic shock syndrome after the

introduction of extraordinarily absorbent tampons in the late 1970s, the Food and Drug Administration created absorbency standards for tampons.

Acacia. *See* Gum arabic.

Acetaminophen. A painkiller sold as a single-ingredient analgesic under many brand names, including Tylenol. It is also used with caffeine in general-market combination products such as Excedrin Extra Strength Caplets and Tablets, and special "women's products" such as Midol PMS, meant for the relief of menstrual cramps. In all cases, acetaminophen is used as a substitute for aspirin or the stronger nonsteroidal anti-inflammatories, often described with the acronym NSAIDs. Unlike aspirin and NSAIDs, acetaminophen does not cause gastric bleeding. However, it lacks the ability to relieve inflammation, and it has side effects of its own. Overdoses may cause nausea, vomiting, chills, and drowsiness; larger overdoses may cause death from liver or kidney damage. Recent studies suggest that taking acetaminophen on an empty stomach may potentiate its side effects.

Acetic acid. A natural preservative and the active ingredient in vinegar. For centuries, acetic acid (in the form of vinegar) has been used as an ingredient in vaginal douches. Today, it is used in brand name commercial douches theoretically to protect against infection by lowering the pH of the vagina, thus making it more acidic to encourage the growth of resident friendly organisms. There is no solid scientific evidence to prove that washing the vagina with a vinegar solution actually accomplishes this.

Acidifying agent, acidifier. An ingredient that increases the acidity of a product or body part. Acetic acid and lactic acid are common acidifiers.

Agar. An emulsifier *(gl.)*, stabilizer *(gl.)*, and thickener derived from seaweed. It is found in cosmetic creams and lotions as well as thickened foods such as jellies and ice cream. It is also used as a bulk producer in laxatives and appetite suppressants.

Alcohol. A synonym for ethyl alcohol *(gl.)*. *See* also Denatured alcohol.

Allergic sensitizer. A chemical that makes people sensitive to other chemicals.

Alginic acid. A hydrophilic ("water loving") substance obtained from seaweed that can absorb up to several hundred times its weight in water and salts. It is used as a suspending agent *(gl.)* and as a bulk producer in laxatives and diet products.

Alkalizer. An ingredient that makes a product more basic (alkaline).

Alkyl-. The word means "derived from alcohol." Ingredients whose name begins with "alkyl" are surfactants and wetting agents generally used in shampoos. *Alkyl aryl sulfonate* and *alkyl sodium sulfonate* are examples of this class of ingredient.

Aloe vera. A natural soothing agent derived from the aloe plant. Fresh aloe juice will deteriorate quickly unless it is chemically treated, so it is purified and "stabilized" for use in cosmetic and drug products. Despite anecdotal evidence, its effectiveness has not yet been established.

Alum. An astringent whose use in vaginal products dates back at least as far as Cleopatra's time. Alum makes tissues swell slightly, causing a tingling sensation. In ancient times it was used in an attempt to restore virginal tightness to the mature vagina; today, its effects are often described in product advertising as a "fresh feeling." Contrary to myth, alum will not shrink the vagina.

Aluminum hydroxide. A basic (alkaline) ingredient used as an astringent in dusting powders, including medicated and antifungal products. In much stronger concentrations, aluminum hydroxide functions as a bleach in hair lighteners for face and body. Strongly concentrated aluminum hydroxide may burn or blister skin; the concentrations in OTC powders are nonirritating. The concentrations in bleaches are safe when used as directed.

Ammonium alum. *See* Alum

Analgesics. Mild painkillers. The term applies to single ingredients such as aspirin, acetaminophen, or ibuprofen, as well as combination products such as Anacin and Midol.

Anionic surfactant. A surfactant/detergent whose molecules carry a negative electric charge. All anionic surfactants are potentially irritating to skin and mucous membranes.

Annatto. A nontoxic, yellow-to-pink vegetable dye used in foods, drugs, and cosmetics.

Antifungal. An ingredient that kills or inhibits the growth of fungi including those that cause vaginal itch.

Anti-inflammatory agent. A chemical that calms the immune system so as to alleviate swelling or redness at the site of an external injury, including an insect bite or another allergic reaction.

Antioxidant. An ingredient that preserves other ingredients, preventing them from combining with oxygen.

Antiseptic. An ingredient that eliminates disease-bearing organisms.

Appetite suppressant. A chemical that reduces the feeling of hunger.

Aromatic oil. A natural substance used to impart fragrance. Aromatic oils may cause a variety of allergic reactions, including photosensitivity (heightened sensitivity to sunlight). Fragrances are the one category in which cosmetic and drug manufacturers do not have to list the actual ingredients on the label; it is enough to write "fragrances" or "aromatic oils."

Aspartame. A synthetic sweetener made from aspartic acid and phenylalanine that has 200 times the sweetness of a comparable amount of table sugar (sucrose). Degrades when heated; may be hazardous to people sensitive to phenylalanine.

Aspirin. A common analgesic whose effectiveness is accepted but has never been subjected to scientific evaluation. Aspirin is not without side effects. It may cause a variety of allergic reactions, including skin rashes and respiratory problems. It can cause gastric bleeding, particularly in people with ulcers or in older people whose stomach lining has thinned with age. If taken within two days before a test for occult (hidden) blood in the stool, aspirin may produce a false positive result. Aspirin is an anticoagulant: it may reduce the risk of heart attack by preventing blood clots, but it can cause hemorrhaging if taken before surgery, including dental surgery. Vitamin C makes aspirin more potent by slowing its elimination from the body. It may also interact with a number of prescription drugs.

Astringent. An ingredient that irritates tissues slightly, may cause them to swell, and produces a prickly or tingling sensation.

B

Baking soda (sodium bicarbonate). A basic (alkaline) ingredient used to raise the pH of a product, making it less acid and more basic. Baking soda is also a natural surfactant *(gl.)* and detergent. It is used in douches and a number of OTC products, including underarm deodorant and body powder.

Base. The fundamental ingredient in a cosmetic or drug product, the one to which the others are added. For example, wax is the base for lipsticks; cornstarch is the base for many dusting powders. Another word for the base in liquid products is "vehicle."

Beeswax. A natural nontoxic wax used as a base for many ointments and creams. Beeswax may be either white or yellow; the yellow has a definite honey fragrance.

Benzethonium chloride. A quaternary ammonium *(gl.)* compound; a cationic surfactant *(gl.)*. Closely related to benzalkonium chloride.

Benzocaine. A topical anesthetic used in anti-itch creams, ointments, and sprays.

Benzoic acid. A preservative and antifungal. Benzoic acid is mildly irritating. It has not been proven safe or effective.

Benzyl alcohol. A constituent of jasmine, hyacinth, and ylang ylang oils, used as a fragrance and antimicrobial. In veterinary medicine, benzyl alcohol has been used to alleviate itching.

Betaine. A nontoxic coloring agent obtained from beets.

Boric acid. An antiseptic *(gl.)*, astringent *(gl.)*, and antifungal ingredient found in several OTC products such as douches. In 1992, the Food and Drug Administration released a report saying that there is insufficient evidence to show that boric acid is effective in OTC products. It may be absorbed into the body through mucous membranes or damaged skin. In high concentrations, this can lead to borate poisoning. Because infants are more sensitive to this than adults, boric acid is no longer used in diaper rash products. The concentrations in douches are presumed to be safe. Note: The symptoms of borate poisoning include central nervous system damage and gastric upset (nausea, vomiting, diarrhea).

Butylparaben. A preservative related to methylparaben and propylparaben. Butylparaben protects products from fungal contamination. It is considered nontoxic, although it may be irritating to skin and mucous membranes.

C

Caffeine. An alkaloid (medication derived from plants); a central nervous system stimulant and mild diuretic found in coffee beans, mate leaves, and the cola nuts used to flavor cola drinks. There are smaller amounts of caffeine in tea leaves, which also contain theine, a similar alkaloid. Cocoa beans contain caffeine plus the muscle stimulant theobromine. There are approximately 100 to 150 mg caffeine in a cup of regular coffee, 60 to 75 mg in a cup of brewed tea, 36 mg in a 6-ounce glass of regular cola, and 3 to 5 mg in a cup of decaffeinated coffee. Caffeine is sometimes added to OTC analgesic products such as Anacin to provide a "lift," and its diuretic action makes it a natural for OTC products designed to relieve PMS.

Calcium carbonate (Chalk). An absorbent powder that occurs naturally in limestone, marble, and coral. Calcium carbonate is used as a base *(gl.)*, a filler, and a thickener. It is virtually nontoxic, an excellent antacid, and a good source of dietary calcium (Tums) for women wishing to maintain bone density as they grow older. Taken in high doses, it may be constipating. Caution: Calcium carbonate may inhibit the body's absorption of tetracyclines. If your doctor has prescribed this antibiotic, check with him or her before using a calcium supplement.

Calcium caseinate. A form of casein, the main protein in cows' milk.

Calcium pantothenate (D-Calcium pantothenate). A dietary supplement sometimes found in diet or nutritional products.

Calcium sulfate. A fine white powder used to thicken foods.

Calcium undecylenate. *See* Undecylenic acid.

Candida albicans, homeopathically prepared. A specially diluted preparation of the fungus linked to vaginal itch and irritation; used in a homeopathic anti-itch product.

Caprylic/capric triglyceride. A mixture of glycerin plus caprylic and capric acids used either as a vehicle *(gl.)* or an emollient *(gl.)*.

Carbomer 934p, carbomer 940 (Carbopol). A thickener, a suspending agent *(gl.)*, a dispersant *(gl.)*, and an emulsifier *(gl.)* used to prevent oils and water from separating. No known toxicity.

Carnauba wax. A potentially allergenic wax from a South American tree. Used to coat tablets and as a texturizer.

Carrageenan (Irish moss). A stabilizer and emulsifier derived from seaweed and used in foods, drugs, and cosmetics.

Casein (Ammonium caseinate, calcium caseinate, potassium caseinate, sodium caseinate). The major protein in cows' milk; used in diet and appetite suppressant products. Nutritious and nontoxic, but may cause allergic reactions in people sensitive to milk and milk products.

Cationic surfactants. A group of surfactants *(gl.)* whose molecules carry a positive electric charge. Cationic surfactants such as benzethonium chloride are quaternary ammonium compounds *(gl.)* used as antiseptics and antimicrobials in household products, cosmetics, and OTC drugs.

Cayenne. Pepper; contains an essential oil that irritates the bladder. Sometimes used as a diuretic.

Cellulose gel. A complex carbohydrate used as a source of dietary fiber in formula diet products and as a bulking agent, an ingredient that makes a product taste fuller.

Cellulose gum (Carboxymethyl cellulose). A synthetic, nontoxic gum derived from cellulose. Used as a thickener in OTC drug products and as a bulk producer (an ingredient that absorbs water but is not absorbed by the body) in appetite suppressants to create a feeling of fullness that encourages the dieter to avoid food.

Cetalkonium chloride. A cationic surfactant *(gl.)* and quaternary ammonium compound *(gl.)* used as a preservative and an antifungal ingredient in OTC drug products and cosmetics.

Cetylpyridinium. An antimicrobial surfactant *(gl.)*, detergent, and quaternary ammonium compound *(gl.)* used as a preservative in OTC drug products such as douche liquids and powders.

Chlorhexidine gluconate. An antiseptic used in feminine deodorant sprays. May irritate skin and mucous membranes.

Chocolate liquor. The liquid product obtained from chocolate beans.

Choline bitartrate. A syrupy liquid; a member of the vitamin B family. Used in formula diet products as a supplement.

Cinnamon powder. A flavoring agent that, like cayenne, may be irritating.

Citric acid. An acid derived from citrus fruits and widely used in foods, drugs, and cosmetics. An acidifier used in OTC douches to lower their pH so as to encourage the growth of "friendly" bacteria in the vagina.

Clotrimazole. An antifungal ingredient, once available only by prescription, now approved for use in OTC products to treat vaginitis and other fungal infections.

Colloidal oatmeal. A form of oatmeal that disperses in water. A natural drying agent and skin soother used in baths to relieve itching from certain rashes. Not for itching caused by dry skin; it will intensify discomfort.

Corn bran. A natural dietary fiber used in formula diet products.

Cornstarch. A powder base used in dusting powders as a substitute for talc.

Counterirritant. An ingredient that, when rubbed on the skin, causes small blood vessels under the surface to dilate so that more blood flows to the tiny blood vessels just under the skin and the skin reddens and feels warmer.

Croscarmellose sodium. A form of cellulose gum; a thickener.

Cystine. A nonessential amino acid; a nutrient found in supplements and diet products.

D

D&C. A prefix used in the names of coloring agents. The initials stand for *drugs* and *cosmetics,* signifying that the agent is considered safe for external use.

Dandelion root. A natural diuretic used in some weight loss tablets.

Denaturant. A chemical added to alcohol, generally ethyl alcohol (ethanol), to make it smell and taste bad.

Denatured alcohol. Alcohol, generally ethyl alcohol (ethanol), to which a denaturant has been added so that the product cannot be used as a beverage. *See also* Ethyl alcohol.

Dextrose. A natural sweetener; a sugar obtained from the corn plant.

Diazolidinyl urea. A relatively new preservative that may be an allergic sensitizer *(gl.).* There is some evidence to suggest that diazolidinyl urea releases formaldehyde, a notorious allergic sensitizer.

Dibasic sodium phosphate. A sequestrant *(gl.),* emulsifier *(gl.),* and alkali-zer *(gl.).* If swallowed, causes purging; sometimes used in laxatives.

Dioctyl sodium sulfosuccinate. An anionic surfactant *(gl.)* used as an emulsifier *(gl.),* a dispersant *(gl.),* and a wetting agent *(gl.)* in a variety of products including vaginal douches. A safe, effective detergent, generally considered nontoxic.

Disodium EDTA (Edetate disodium). A sequestrant; attracts and inactivates the calcium ions required by *Trichomonas vaginitis* organisms; not proven safe or effective for relieving minor irritations.

Disodium phosphate. An ingredient used in formula diet products to keep proteins from degenerating, to prevent liquid formula from solidifying, and to balance the acidity in chocolate preparations.

Dispersant. An ingredient that keeps particles of material spread evenly in liquids.

Distilled water. Water that has been purified by boiling. The water is heated to the boiling point, and the steam is re-collected as water. In the process, impurities such as minerals and chemicals are left behind.

Diuretic. An ingredient that increases the body's output of urine.

E

EDTA. *See* Ethylenediaminetetraacetic acid.

Emollient. An oily ingredient that softens the skin.

Emulsifier. An ingredient that makes it possible to mix otherwise unmixable liquids such as oil and water. Emulsifiers create a liquid-in-liquid emulsion, a common formulation for cosmetics and OTC drug products.

Ergocalciferol (Vitamin D2). A nutrient included in diet products and vitamin supplements.

Ethanol. *See* Ethyl alcohol.

Ethinyl estradiol. A synthetic estrogen used in birth control pills.

Ethyl alcohol (Alcohol, ethanol). Ordinary grain alcohol, often written simply as "alcohol." Ethyl alcohol is a solvent *(gl.)* in cosmetics, OTC drugs, and household products, often as denatured alcohol *(gl.)*.

Ethylcellulose. Fiber used as a filler in pills and tablets.

Ethylenediaminetetraacetic acid (Edetate, EDTA). A water softener and sequestrant *(gl.)* that keeps liquid cosmetics and drugs clear of particles by attracting and inactivating microscopic, floating mineral particles.

Ethynodiol diacetate. A progestin (synthetic progesterone) used in birth control pills.

Eucalyptus oil. An essential oil from eucalyptus leaves. Used as a fragrance, counterirritant, and preservative in OTC drug products. It may cause allergic reactions in sensitive people. Pure eucalyptus oil is toxic. As little as seven drops taken by mouth may be fatal.

F

Fatty acids. Acids derived from animal or vegetable fat; used to make soaps.

FD&C. A prefix used in the names of artificial (synthetic) coloring agents. The initials stand for *food, drugs,* and *cosmetics,* meaning the ingredient is considered safe for external and internal use.

Ferric ammonium citrate, ferric fumarate, ferrous gluconate, ferrous sulfate. See Iron sources.

Fine silica. See Silica, Silica (fine).

Fructose. A natural sweetener obtained from fruits.

G

Gluconodeltalactone. A sequestrant *(gl.)*; keeps liquids clear by attracting and inactivating mineral particles.

Glycerides. The major constituents of animal and vegetable fats and oils; used as emulsifiers to keep the ingredients in the product from separating. Glycerides are created through a reaction between glycerol and fatty acids. The prefixes mono-, di-, or tri- in front of the word *glyceride* describes the ratio of glycerol to fatty acids. Glycerides may be saturated or unsaturated fats.

Glycerol, glycerin, glycerine. A sweet-smelling fat found in animal and plant oils and fats; separated from fat as a by-product in the manufacture of soap. Glycerol is used as a humectant *(gl.)*, an emollient *(gl.)*, and a base or thickener in oily products such as suppositories. It is nontoxic and soothing to the skin but may irritate mucous membranes.

Glyceryl monostearate (Monostearin). A nontoxic white, waxy, solid material combined with soap to act as a surfactant or emulsifier.

Guar gum (Jaguar gum). A natural thickener obtained from *Cyamopsis tetragonolobus,* which is cultivated in India as feed for livestock. Guar gum has five to six times the thickening power of starches.

Gum arabic. A sticky substance from the bark of the acacia tree, which grows in the American South, the Near East, Africa, and India. Gum arabic is used as a thickener in contraceptive jellies and creams. It is also a food additive, a stabilizer that keeps bubbles and foam from disappearing too quickly from beer and soft drinks, a thickener in jellies and jams, and a natural emulsifier used to keep ingredients in liquid products such as formula diet drinks from separating.

Gum tragacanth (Tragacanth). The gummy exudate of an Asian shrub, *Astragalus gummifer,* used as an emulsifier *(gl.)*. It is odorless and very sticky. It is generally nontoxic by mouth but may cause allergic reactions in sensitive people who touch or swallow it.

H

HCG. An abbreviation for human chorionic gonadotropin, a hormone secreted by the membrane surrounding the fetus in the womb. HCG is the hormone detected by pregnancy tests.

HCG antiserum (Anti-HCG). Antibodies that react in the presence of HCG; the active ingredient in pregnancy test kits.

Histidine. An amino acid used as a nutrient in diet products.

Horsetail. A mildly diuretic herb.

Humectant. A thick, syrupy liquid that attracts and holds moisture. Humectants are used to prevent products from drying out.

Hydrangea. An ingredient from the dried rhizomes and roots of *Hydrangea arborescens*. A reputed diuretic, sometimes included in products to relieve the symptoms of PMS.

Hydrocortisone. An anti-inflammatory, anti-itch drug once available only by prescription, now included in OTC products such as products to relieve vaginal itch.

Hydrogenated palm oil. An oil from the fruit or seed of the palm tree that has been hardened via the addition of hydrogen atoms. Used as an emollient in OTC drugs.

Hydrogenated vegetable oil. An oil, such as corn oil or palm oil, derived from a vegetable and hardened through the addition of hydrogen atoms. Used as an emollient in OTC drugs.

Hydrolyzed silica. *See* Silica.

Hydroxyethylcellulose. An ingredient created through a reaction between cellulose and ethylene oxide. Used as a thickener in cosmetics and drugs.

Hydroxyquinoline. An antifungal with antiseptic and deodorant properties. Used in products to treat vaginal itch.

I

Invert sugar. A 50/50 mixture of glucose and fructose.

Iodine. *See* Povidone-iodine.

Iron oxides. Chemicals created by combining iron with oxygen that are used as dyes.

Iron sources. Nutritional supplements found in diet products and vitamin/mineral preparations, primarily for women of childbearing age, to counter iron-deficiency anemia. In normal doses, iron is not considered toxic for adults. However, iron poisoning from iron supplements is not uncommon among small children who mistake the pills for candy. In October 1994, the Food and Drug Administration proposed regulations to require warning labels on iron products containing more than 30 mg iron in each dose (pill, tablet, teaspoon, etc.). The proposal is based on the fact that drugs and supplements containing iron are the leading cause of accidental poisoning among children. From 1988 to 1992, nearly 20 percent of all children's deaths reported to poison control centers in the United States were due to iron poisoning. The lethal doses ranged from as few as 5 tablets to as many as 98.

Isobutane. A flammable propellant gas used in OTC aerosol products such as anti-itch sprays. Inhalation of concentrated vapors may cause unconsciousness.

Isopropyl alcohol (Isopropanol, 2-propanol). A flammable liquid that smells like a cross between alcohol and acetone, the solvent used in nail polish removers. An antiseptic and counterirritant found in a variety of drug and cosmetic products. It makes the skin feel tingly and stings mucous membranes. If swallowed or if concentrated vapors are inhaled, it can cause intoxication: flushed skin, headache, dizziness, mental depression, nausea, and vomiting. In large amounts, it is potentially fatal.

Isopropyl myristate. An emollient also used as a solvent for waxes and fats. It may irritate skin and mucous membranes, and it is an allergic sensitizer *(gl.)*.

J

Jaguar gum. *See* Guar gum.

Juniper berries. The dried, ripe fruit of *Juniperus communis,* which grows in North America, northern Europe, and Asia, a primary flavoring agent in gin. The essential oil is a diuretic.

K

Kaolin. A clay (hydrated aluminum silicate) used in poultices and in Kaopectate, a brand name antidiarrheal. It is nontoxic, but if swallowed in large quantities without sufficient liquids, it may solidify and obstruct the intestines.

L

Lactic acid. An acidifier; often used in OTC douche solutions to make them more acidic to lower the pH of the vaginal tissues and to encourage the growth of "friendly" bacteria. There is virtually no scientific evidence to show that acidic douche solutions produce long-term effects on vaginal pH.

Lactobacilli. *See* Yogurt.

Lactose. The primary sugar in milk and a bacterial nutrient included in OTC douche solutions to encourage the growth of "friendly" bacteria in the vagina.

Lanolin alcohol. A solid, waxy material made from lanolin (the oil in sheep's wool) and used as an emulsifier and emollient.

Laureth 23. Detergent/surfactant produced from coconut oil. May be mildly irritating to skin and mucous membranes.

Lecithin. A nutritional supplement included in some liquid diet products and appetite suppressants as an emulsifier to keep the ingredients from separating.

Levonorgestrel. A synthetic progesterone used in birth control pills and for menopausal hormone replacement therapy.

M

Magnesium chloride. An ingredient used in products to retain color and firmness.

Magnesium hydroxide. An alkaline powder used as a skin soother.

Magnesium oxide. *See* Magnesium hydroxide.

Magnesium phosphate. A mineral supplement in nutritional products.

Magnesium stearate. A nontoxic, white powder used as a filler in tablets and a skin soother in dusting powders.

Malt extract. A barley extract used as a nutrient in formula diet products.

Maltodextrin. A texturizer *(gl.)* and flavor enhancer created from cornstarch. Used to "bulk up" liquid diet formula foods.

Menthol. An aromatic chemical obtained from oil of peppermint. It is a topical anesthetic that produces a tingly feeling on skin and mucous membranes. It is also used as a perfume and a preservative. Its safety and effectiveness as an astringent remain to be proven.

Mestranol. A synthetic estrogen used in birth control pills.

1-methionine. An essential amino acid used in vitamin/mineral and formula diet supplements.

Methylbenzethonium chloride. A quaternary ammonium compound used as a topical germicide and disinfectant. Derived from Benzethonium chloride.

Methylcellulose. A semi-synthetic derivative of cellulose that absorbs and holds large amounts of water. It is nontoxic, but if taken without sufficient quantities of liquid, it may solidify and obstruct the intestines.

Methylparaben. A preservative, antifungal, and antibacterial. Nontoxic when fed to laboratory animals in amounts up to 8 percent of the total diet. Unlikely to be irritating or to act as an allergic sensitizer *(gl.)* although it may cause allergic reactions in some sensitive individuals.

Methyl salicylate (Betula oil, oil of wintergreen, sweet birch oil). An aromatic oil derived from the leaves of the sweet birch, cassia, or wintergreen. An antiseptic, a preservative, and a counterirritant *(gl.)*. Persons allergic to aspirin may be allergic to methyl salicylate. When rubbed on the skin, it may cause photosensitivity (unusual sensitivity to sunlight). It may also be absorbed through the skin.

Miconazole. An antifungal ingredient used to treat *Candida albicans* vaginitis. The crystalline part of cellulose fibers.

Mineral oil (Liquid petrolatum, white oil). A mixture of refined, liquid hydrocarbons derived from petroleum. Mineral oil is a first cousin to petroleum jelly, a solid hydrocarbon compound. Colorless, flavorless, odorless, and nontoxic, but acts as a laxative if swallowed in large amounts. It is used in a variety of oily products.

Monoamine oxidase inhibitors (MAO inhibitors). Antidepressant drugs.

Monobasic sodium phosphate. An acidifier used to lower the pH *(gl.)* of solutions, that is, to make them more acidic.

N

Nonionic surfactant. A surfactant *(gl.)* whose molecules carry neither a positive nor a negative electric charge.

Nonoxynol-9 (Nonylphenoxypolyethoxyethanol). A surfactant used as a spermicide in contraceptive jellies, creams, and foams.

Norethindrone. A synthetic form of the female sex hormone progesterone. Used in birth control pills.

Norgestimate. A synthetic form of the female sex hormone progesterone. Used in birth control pills.

Norgestrel. A synthetic form of the female sex hormone progesterone. Used in birth control pills.

NSAIDs (Nonsteroidal anti-inflammatory drugs). A class of analgesics *(gl.)* that relieve pain and inflammation without the side effects associated with steroid hormones.

O

Octoxynol-9. A nonionic surfactant/detergent used in spermicides and other products. Despite long use and anecdotal evidence of effectiveness, octoxynol-9 has not been proven safe or effective as a contraceptive.

Oxyquinoline. *See* Hydroxyquinoline.

P

Pamabrom. A diuretic *(gl.)* found in many OTC products to treat PMS.

PEG. *See* Polyethylene glycols.

pH. Acid/base (alkaline) balance. Acidifiers are used to lower the pH, that is, to make it more acid. Alkalizers are used to raise the pH, that is, to make it more basic (alkaline). An acidic or basic solution may be important in a health product. For example, douche solutions are generally acidic to encourage the growth of "good" bacteria in the vagina.

Phenol. A caustic poison, also known as carbolic acid. Phenol is obtained from coal tar and benzene compounds. It is used, in very low concentrations, as an antiseptic, counterirritant *(gl.)*, and disinfectant in a variety of products, including household cleaners and OTC cosmetics and drugs such as hand lotions. It is toxic if swallowed, even in small amounts, and it may be absorbed through the skin.

Phenylalanine. An essential amino acid, used as a nutrient in some diet products and supplements.

Poloxamers. Nonionic, nontoxic surfactants sometimes used in spermicides. Distinguished from each other by a number, such as Poloxamer 188. The number refers to the ingredient's molecular weight.

Polyethylene glycols. Waxy substances used in a variety of products. Often described with the acronym PEG plus a number (such as PEG-8). The higher the number, the more solid the substance.

Polysorbates. A group of emulsifiers *(gl.)*, stabilizers *(gl.)*, and non-ionic surfactants *(gl.)*. The individual compounds are identified by a number that indicates the ingredient's molecular weight, such as Polysorbate 20.

Potassium sorbate. A preservative that inhibits the growth of molds and yeasts. Widely used in foods; used in vaginal douches for the relief of minor irritation due to yeast infection.

Povidone-iodine. An antimicrobial used in medicated vaginal douches to relieve itch and irritation due to yeast infection.

Powdered cellulose. A complex carbohydrate used to provide dietary fiber and as a bulking agent (to provide "body") for formula diet products.

1,2-propanediol. A synonym for Propylene glycol.

Propylene glycol. A thick, clear, colorless liquid used as a preservative, a mold inhibitor, a humectant *(gl.)*, and a solvent *(gl.)*. May cause allergic reactions in sensitive individuals.

Propylparaben. A preservative and an antifungal ingredient, related to butylparaben and methylparaben.

Psyllium seed husks (Plantago seed). A laxative.

Pulsitilla (Pasque flower, wind flower, meadow anemone). Dried herb used in homeopathic medicine for a variety of ills. Patch tests show that it may cause allergic reactions, including blisters and pigmentation of skin at test site; vapors may be irritating.

Purified water. A synonym for distilled water *(gl.)*.

Pyrilamine Maleate. An antihistamine sometimes used as a mild sedative, as in products designed to alleviate the symptoms of PMS or menstrual discomfort.

Q

Quaternary ammonium compounds. Cationic surfactants widely used as sanitizers and deodorizers. They are often described with the word *quaternium* followed by a number, such as quaternium-1 and quaternium-2. These compounds are relatively safe in low concentrations. In high concentrations, however, they may be severely irritating to skin and mucous membranes and potentially lethal if swallowed. (The possible lethal dose for an adult is 1 teaspoon.)

R

Rayon. Either a fiber made from cellulose (which comes from wood) or any thread, yarn, or material made from those fibers. Rayon is used in sanitary napkins and tampons. It may (rarely) cause an allergic skin rash.

Resorcinol. An antiseptic, preservative, and astringent used in some anti-itch products. Paradoxically, resorcinol may be severely irritating to skin and mucous membranes.

Retinol, retinoic acid. *See* Vitamin A.

Riboflavin (Vitamin B2). A nutrient found in supplements as well as some diet products. Riboflavin assists in the metabolism of sugars and starches and helps maintain the integrity and health of the skin. Symptoms of a riboflavin deficiency include sore or cracked lips, skin blemishes, and vision problems.

S

Saponins. Sugar and alcohol compounds that occur naturally in plants and are nontoxic to human beings. They foam in water and are used in making soaps and detergents. They may also be used as emulsifiers.

SD alcohol. A denatured alcohol *(gl.)* used as a thickener or liquefier. The name of each ingredient product includes a number, such as SD Alcohol 40.

Sequestering agent. Keeps liquids clear by attracting and precipitating free-floating microscopic metal particles.

Silica (Sodium dioxide). A mineral that occurs in nature as agate, amethyst, flint, quartz, and sand.

Silica (fine). Ground silica used in powders to make them pour more smoothly. However, even fine silica is abrasive and may be irritating to skin or mucous membranes.

Silicon. The second most abundant element on earth after oxygen, silicon comprises about 28 percent of the earth's crust.

Silicon dioxide. A synonym for silica.

Silicon oil. A silicone.

Silicones. Lubricants and waterproofers manufactured from silicon and oxygen compounds called siloxanes. Silicones occur in many forms, including resins and oils. They are sometimes used as lubricants on latex condoms.

Simethicone. A silicone oil; a thick white liquid used as a base for ointments and gels such as contraceptives jellies.

Soap. A basic (alkaline), natural cleanser; a mixture of animal or vegetable fat and an alkali (lye). Modern toilet soaps often include humectants *(gl.)* and oils. Unlike detergents, which are synthetic cleansers, soaps leave a residue of scum on skin and hair. Before the introduction of detergent-based shampoos, acids such as vinegar and lemon juice were commonly used as rinses to remove the basic (alkaline) soap scum from hair.

Sodium acetate. An alkalizer used to stabilize the pH (acid/base balance) in cosmetic and drug products.

Sodium ascorbate. A form of vitamin C; an antioxidant *(gl.)*.

Sodium benzoate. A preservative and antimicrobial.

Sodium bicarbonate. A synonym for baking soda.

Sodium carboxymethylcellulose (CMC, carboxymethyl cellulose sodium). A nontoxic, artificial gum produced from cellulose. Used as a suspending agent *(gl.)*, a thickener, and a bulk producer (an ingredient that absorbs water but is not absorbed by the body) in appetite suppressants to create a feeling of fullness, which encourages the dieter to avoid food.

Sodium caseinate. A powder derived from cows' milk that is used as a texturizer *(gl.)*.

Sodium chloride (Salt, table salt). An antiseptic *(gl.)* and an astringent *(gl.)*; may be drying to the skin or mucous membranes.

Sodium edetate (Sodium EDTA, sodium salt of ethylenediaminetetra-acidic acid, tetra sodium edetate, tetra EDTA). A sequestering agent *(gl.)* that keeps liquids clear by attracting and precipitating free-floating microscopic metal particles.

Sodium hydroxide (Caustic soda, lye). An alkali that is used in very weak concentrations as an emulsifier in soaps and creams.

Sodium lactate. A thick, colorless, odorless liquid used as an acidifier in vaginal douches and as a plasticizer (thickener) in a variety of products.

Sodium lauryl sulfate (Dodecyl sodium sulfate). One of a group of anionic surfactants with the generic name *sodium lauryl sulfates*. A wetting agent and detergent used in vaginal douche products to increase the liquid's ability to spread out and cover vaginal tissues and to help flush out secretions.

Sodium propionate. A preservative, an antifungal, and a mold inhibitor.

Sodium silicate (soluble glass). An anticaking agent that keeps powdered drug and cosmetic products from clumping in the package. May be irritating to skin and mucous membranes; causes gastric upset if swallowed.

Solvent. An ingredient that dissolves other ingredients. Water is the most common solvent.

Sorbic acid (2,4-Hexadienoic acid). A mold and yeast inhibitor as well as a humectant *(gl.)*. May cause skin irritation in sensitive people.

Sorbitan monostearate (Sorbitan stearate). A humectant created through a reaction between fatty acids and sorbitol *(gl.)*. Used in creams and lotions. Nontoxic and edible, but consuming large amounts may cause diarrhea.

Sorbitol. A natural product derived from the ripe berries of the mountain ash, *Pyrus aucuparia,* as well as from many other berries, fruits, and plants such as cherries, plums, pears, apples, seaweed, and algae. Sorbitol is a natural sweetener, absorbed more slowly than table sugar. It is also a humectant *(gl.)*. It is nontoxic in normal amounts; when taken in excess, it can cause gastric upset, primarily diarrhea.

Soy fiber. A form of fiber used in formula diet foods.

Soy lecithin. Lecithin from soybeans. *See also* Lecithin.

Soy protein isolate. Protein from soybeans, used in formula diet products.

Spermaceti. A nontoxic, odorless, flavorless, waxy substance from the head of the sperm whale. Used as a base in emollients, ointments, and suppositories.

Stabilizer. An ingredient that keeps the components of emulsions (*see* Emulsifier) from separating.

Starch. A carbohydrate that occurs naturally in corn, potatoes, rice, tapioca, and other plants. Forms a stiff gel when combined with warm liquids. Sometimes used in aerosol foam products such as contraceptive foams to keep the foam from breaking down too quickly.

Stearic acid (Octadecanoic acid). A nontoxic glyceride *(gl.)* from animal fats. Used in creams, lotions, and foams, as well as hardened-oil products such as suppositories.

Sucrose. A natural sweetener; table sugar.

Surfactant. A substance that increases a product's cleansing abilities. Surfactants are sometimes called "wetting agents" because they allow liquids to spread out faster and cover more surface. *See also* Anionic surfactant, Cationic surfactant, Nonionic surfactant.

Suspending agent. An ingredient that keeps particles of other ingredients evenly spread out in a liquid, producing a stable product.

T

Talc (Talcum). Finely powdered magnesium silicate, a mineral found in the earth's crust. Once universal in body powders. Because particles of talc were found in some ovarian and cervical tumors, talc is no longer used in vaginal dusting powders. It may still be found in body powders and in some medicated powders used to treat fungal infections of the groin area.

Tartaric acid. A fruit acid and a by-product of wine-making. Sometimes used as an acidifier to maintain the pH (acid/base balance) of OTC products.

Tetramethylbenzidine. The active ingredient in self-tests for occult blood in the stool.

Texturizer. A chemical that improves texture, for example, preventing lumps in creams and lotions.

Thickener. An ingredient that makes products more viscous or stiff.

Thymol. A preservative, an antifungal, a mold and mildew inhibitor, and a counterirritant. If swallowed, it may cause nausea, vomiting, convulsions, and coma. The probable lethal dose for an adult is 1 teaspoon of pure thymol.

Titanium dioxide. A white powder used as a pigment to make dusting powder and other powder products white and opaque.

Tolnaftate. An antifungal and the most popular active ingredient in medicated OTC powders, ointments, creams, and sprays to treat athlete's foot and fungal infections of the groin.

Tricalcium phosphate. An anticaking ingredient used to keep drug and cosmetic powders from clumping.

Triethanolamine (TEA). A thick, viscous liquid with a faint smell of ammonia. Also an emulsifier (gl.) that forms a soap when combined with fatty acids.

Triethanolamine dodecylbenzene sulfonate. An emulsifier *(gl.)* and surfactant *(gl.)*. May be irritating to skin and mucous membranes.

U

Undecylenic acid. An antifungal (gl.), antibacterial ingredient considered effective against *Candida albicans*. Often used in products (powders, creams, ointments) to combat external vaginal itch. Its unusual odor, which some say resembles sweat or urine, is usually masked by fragrance. Other forms are calcium undecylenate and zinc undecylenate.

Urea. An antiseptic, deodorizer, diuretic *(gl.)*, and skin-soothing humectant *(gl.)* found in a wide variety of OTC drug and cosmetic products, particularly hand and body lotions.

Uva ursi (Bearberry). The dried leaves of *Arctostaphylos uva ursi,* which grows in northern Europe, North America, and Asia. A urinary antiseptic sometimes used as a diuretic in OTC products to relieve the symptoms of PMS.

V

Vegetable oil base. Any of a number of oils derived from plants and used as vehicles *(gl.)* for cosmetic and OTC drug products. Cocoa butter is a common vegetable oil base, widely used in vaginal and rectal suppositories. Nontoxic and edible, but may cause allergic reactions in sensitive individuals.

Vehicle. A liquid used as a base *(gl.)* for a product such as a douche or lotion.

Vinegar. *See* Acetic acid.

Vitamin A (Retinol). A nutrient included in diet products and nutritional supplements. Sometimes included in hand and body lotions; alleged to heal and soothe skin. Retinoic acid, a derivative of vitamin A, helps slough dead cells off the skin surface and is widely used in "rejuvenating" creams and lotions.

W

Water. The primary solvent *(gl.)* and vehicle *(gl.)* used in OTC drugs and cosmetics. *See* Purified water.

Wax. A "thermoplastic" material—soft and pliable when warm, hard and brittle when cold—used in oily products such as suppositories and ointments. Waxes occur widely in nature, produced by animals (beeswax) or derived from minerals (ceresin, mineral oil, ozokerite). They are generally nontoxic; if swallowed, they act as laxatives.

Wetting agent. A surfactant *(gl.)*.

Whey powder. A powder made from the liquid part of milk that remains when the solid casein *(gl.)* has been removed.

X

Xanthan gum. A thick, gummy liquid produced by the bacterium *Xanthomonas campestris* and converted to a cream-colored, odorless powder that dissolves easily in water. It is used as an emulsifier and stabilizer in foods, drugs, and cosmetics.

Xylitol. A natural sweetener, equal to sugar in sweetening power but without sugar's ability to trigger cavities.

Y

Yeast. Moist or dried living cells of fungi. Sometimes used in nutritional supplements as a source of vitamin B complex.

Yogurt, yogurt culture. A source of lactobacilli, bacteria that normally live in the healthy vagina. Sometimes included in douche preparations.

Z

Zea (Cornsilk). Dried material from corn plants (*Zea mays*) sometimes included as a diuretic ingredient in products designed to relieve symptoms of PMS.

Zinc oxide. An astringent and an opacifier used primarily as a color (whitening) agent in powders, ointments, and lotions. May irritate the skin.

Zinc sulfate. An astringent; a source of dietary zinc.

Zinc undecylenate. *See* Undecylenic acid.

SOURCES

Duke, James A., *Handbook of Medicinal Herbs* (Boca Raton, FL: CRC Press, 1988).

"Iron toxicity warning," *FDA Medical Bulletin,* February 1995.

Gosselin, Robert E., et al., *Clinical Toxicology of Commercial Products* (Baltimore, MD: Williams and Wilkins, 1976).

Long, James W., and James Rybacki, *The Essential Guide to Prescription Drugs 1995* (New York: HarperCollins, 1995).

Martin, Eric W., *The Hazards of Medication* (Philadelphia: J.B. Lippincott, 1978).

The Merck Index, 11th ed. (Rahway, NJ: Merck & Co., 1989).

Registry of Toxic Effects of Chemical Substances (National Institute for Occupational Safety and Health, 1979).

Rinzler, Carol Ann, *Strictly Female* (New York: New American Library, 1981).

Winter, Ruth, *A Consumer's Dictionary of Cosmetic Ingredients*, 4th ed. (New York: Crown Publishers, 1994).

INDEX

[Names of trademarked products are indicated by an initial capital letter.]

WOMEN'S HEALTH & SEXUALITY

THE NEW A-TO-Z OF WOMEN'S HEALTH: A Concise Encyclopedia
by Christine Ammer

This essential reference puts the very latest information on over 1000 health topics at women's fingertips. From contraceptives to osteoporosis, from patient's rights to the symptoms of depression, each subject is covered in clear, jargon-free language, in both clinical and real-life terms, supported by charts, diagrams, and an appendix of resources. All entries are cross-referenced to quickly answer a wide range of health questions covering drugs and disabilities; common tests and procedures; cholesterol and diet; breast disease and sexuality; medications, and vitamins.

> **"On your bookshelf next to *Our Bodies, Our Selves,* you can now put Christine Ammer's *The New A-to-Z of Women's Health*."** — *Ms.*

496 pages ... 10 illus. ... Paperback ... $16.95

FROM ACUPRESSURE TO ZEN: An Encyclopedia of Natural Therapies
by Barbara Nash

Natural therapies make a wonderful complement to traditional medicine. This book provides clear descriptions of over 70 therapies, from ayurvedic medicine and Bach flower remedies to homeopathy, T'ai Chi, and Zen. Each entry includes information on the therapy's origin, how it helps, and how traditional doctors feel about it. It also lists more than 150 ailments and suggests natural therapies to treat them. Special sections cover pregnancy, family health, and sexuality.

288 pages ... 24 illus. ... Paperback $15.95 ... Hard cover $25.95

WOMEN, SEX & DESIRE: Exploring Your Sexuality at Every Stage of Life
by Elizabeth Davis, with a Foreword by Germaine Greer

A women's sexuality is a synthesis of her emotion, intuition, energy, and spirituality, and it affects all aspects of her life and self. Midwife and author Elizabeth Davis describes the natural cycles of a woman's sexuality, weaving new biological information, descriptions of cultural rituals, and personal stories into a tapestry reflecting women's changing moods, desires, and passions over a lifetime.

> **"Ready to occupy a central place on the women's health bookshelf, this [book is a] comprehensive, quietly authoritative consideration of female sexuality."** — *Publishers Weekly*

224 pages ... 9 illus. ... Paperback $12.95 ... Hard cover $22.95

SEXUAL PLEASURE: Reaching New Heights of Sexual Arousal and Intimacy
by Barbara Keesling, Ph.D.

This bestselling book is for all people who want to discover the key to fulfilling sex: getting in touch with their own sexuality and arousal. This will make them more relaxed and sensitive to their partner's needs, and leads to greater sexual pleasure for both partners. Dr. Keesling offers new ideas and exercises throughout the book, including: **For women:** never-before published methods on how to have orgasms easily using internal and external trigger points. **For men:** exercises to prolong their erections and synchronize orgasm and ejaculation. **For both partners:** creative ways to play together, increase intimacy, and achieve intense mutual arousal.

224 pages ... 14 photographs ... Paperback $12.95 ... Hardcover $21.95

Call for our FREE catalog of books at (800) 266-5592

CHRONIC FATIGUE & WOMEN'S HEALTH

RUNNING ON EMPTY: The Complete Guide to Chronic Fatigue Syndrome (CFIDS)
by Katrina Berne, Ph.D.

Sore throat, fatigue, vertigo, headache, muscle pain, fever, depression — if you are unable to shake these symptoms you may be suffering from from Chronic Fatigue Syndrome. Although it can be difficult to diagnose, CFIDS is a real, biologically-based disease with options for effective treatment and management. Written by an expert who has CFIDS herself, this book offers clarity, hope, and support. It includes summaries of recent medical findings on treatments, ideas on living with the disease, and intimate stories of other sufferers. The accurate information and sympathetic, upbeat tone make this an invaluable book for CFIDS patients and a complete reference for the health care professionals who treat them.

> **"Well-researched, well-organized, and eminently readable, this book should prove quite a boon to CFIDS sufferers."** — *Booklist*

336 pages ... Paperback $14.95 ... Hard cover $24.95 ... 2nd edition

ONCE A MONTH: The Original Premenstrual Syndrome Handbook
by Katharina Dalton, M.D.

Once considered an imaginary complaint, PMS has at last received the serious attention it deserves, thanks largely to the work of Dr. Katharina Dalton. Premenstrual syndrome may in fact be the world's most common condition: surveys show that as many as 75% of women experience at least one symptom. The fifth edition of this classic book covers all the issues including the symptoms, effects, and medical and self-help treatment options.

> **"Dalton is amply qualified to make the diagnosis."** — *Newsweek*

288 pages ... 36 illus. ... Paperback ... $14.95 ... 5th edition

THE FERTILITY AWARENESS HANDBOOK: The Natural Guide to Avoiding or Achieving Pregnancy *by* Barbara Kass-Annese, R.N., and Hal C. Danzer, M.D.

The language of a woman's body tells her the days of the month when she is most fertile and likely to conceive, and when she is infertile and can safely have sex without conceiving. The methods described in this book are based on this language and give women a contraceptive choice or an enhanced opportunity to become pregnant. These scientifically proven methods have no side-effects, no hormone-related dangers. They teach women to be more in touch with their bodies, more secure in the lovemaking, and more in control of their sexual well-being.

160 pages ... 47 illus. ... Paperback ... $11.95

GETTING PREGNANT AND STAYING PREGNANT: Overcoming Infertility and Managing Your High-Risk Pregnancy *by* Diana Raab, R.N.

This is a practical guide to the physical, medical, and emotional issues women and their partners face during infertility treatments and high-risk pregnancies. Winner of the 1992 Benjamin Franklin Award for Best Health Book, it combines accurate medical information with a nurse's thoughtfulness and care. In **Part One,** detailed chapters cover new infertility technologies, tests, and genetic risks. **Part Two** combines information about what to expect during a high-risk pregnancy with supportive ideas for coping with cesareans, miscarriages, and premature babies.

336 pages ... 28 illus. ... Paperback ... $14.95

To order see last page or call (800) 266-5592

MENOPAUSE, SMOKING CESSATION

MENOPAUSE WITHOUT MEDICINE *by* Linda Ojeda, Ph.D.

Linda Ojeda broke new ground when she began her study of nonmedical approaches to menopause more than ten years ago. Now she has fully updated her classic book. She discusses: natural sources of estrogen, including phytoestrogens; how mood swings are affected by diet and personality; and the newest research on osteoporosis, breast cancer, and heart disease. She thoroughly examines the hormone therapy debate; suggests natural remedies for depression, hot flashes, sexual changes, and skin and hair problems; and presents an illustrated basic exercise program. Throughout, Ojeda shows how women can enjoy optimal health at any age with a good diet and nurturing lifestyle. ***As seen in Time magazine.***

352 pages ... 40 illus. ... Paperback $13.95 ... Hard cover $23.95 ... 3rd edition

THE MENOPAUSE INDUSTRY: How the Medical Establishment Exploits Women
by Sandra Coney

Menopause is a natural stage in a woman's life, yet it is treated as a disease, something to fear and medicate. This provocative book shows how menopause myths have been built on incomplete and misquoted research so the healthcare industry can sell products and services.

> **"Read this book and become enraged! Sandra Coney's balanced approach gives information and therefore power back to all midlife women." — Susan Love, M.D., author of** *Dr. Susan Love's Breast Book*

384 pages ... 31 illus. ... Paperback $14.95 ... Hardcover $24.95

ESTROGEN & BREAST CANCER: A Warning to Women *by* Carol Ann Rinzler

From the author of *The Women's Health Products Handbook,* this cautionary tale about American medicine's experimentation with female hormones examines the evidence linking the rise in breast cancer to the increased use of estrogen — especially the Pill and hormone replacement therapy. Rinzler details studies showing estrogen to be a potential carcinogen and, avoiding a blanket condemnation of estrogen, discusses how women can balance the benefits against the risks.

> **"Every woman considering postmenopause hormonal therapy should read this book first and remember that there is no free lunch."—Susan Love, M.D., author of** *Dr. Susan Love's Breast Book*

256 pages ... 12 illus. ... Paperback ... $14.95

HOW WOMEN CAN *FINALLY* STOP SMOKING *by* Robert C. Klesges, Ph.D., and Margaret DeBon, M.S.

Based on Memphis State University's highly acclaimed smoking-cessation program, this book reveals that women start smoking, continue to smoke, and relapse after quitting for different reasons than men. Women's bodies also react to nicotine differently, so withdrawal symptoms are more severe and they gain weight. **Part One** guides women in choosing the best time to quit and the method to use. **Part Two** gives directions for managing withdrawal, finding support, and controlling stress. A key chapter offers three simple strategies to prevent relapse. Includes a pull-out stop-smoking checklist and self-monitoring diary to note the times of day you smoke.

192 pages ... Paperback ... $9.95

Prices subject to change without notice

ORDER FORM

10% DISCOUNT on orders of $20 or more —		
20% DISCOUNT on orders of $50 or more —		
30% DISCOUNT on orders of $250 or more —		
On cost of books for fully prepaid orders		

NAME

ADDRESS

CITY/STATE   ZIP/POSTCODE

PHONE   COUNTRY (outside U.S.)

TITLE	QTY	PRICE	TOTAL
Women's Health Products... (paperback)	|	@ $ 15.95	
Women's Health Products...(hard cover)	|	@ $ 25.95	
List other titles and prices below:			
	|	@ $	
	|	@ $	
	|	@ $	
	|	@ $	
	|	@ $	
	|	@ $	
	|	@ $	
	|	@ $	
	|	@ $	
	|	@ $	

SHIPPING COSTS:
First book: $3.00 by book post ($4.50 by UPS or to ship outside the U.S.)
Each additional book: $1.00
For bulk orders call us at (510) 865-5282

TOTAL	
Less discount @ _____%	(_____)
TOTAL COST OF BOOKS	_____
Calif. residents add sales tax	_____
Shipping & handling	_____
TOTAL ENCLOSED *Please pay in U.S. funds only*	_____

☐ Check   ☐ Money Order   ☐ Visa   ☐ M/C   ☐ Discover

Card # _____ Exp date _____

Signature _____

Complete and mail to:

Hunter House Inc., Publishers
P.O. Box 2914, Alameda CA 94501-0914

Orders: (800) 266-5592   Email: ordering@hunterhouse.com
Phone (510) 865-5282 Fax (510) 865-4295

☐ Check here to receive our FREE book catalog

WHP 12/96